Stories in Health Communication: Reflection, Inquiry, Action

Stories in Health Communication: Reflection, Inquiry, Action

Gjyn O'Toole

ELSEVIER

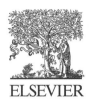

ISBN: 978-0-7295-4456-6

Notice

National Library of Australia Cataloguing-in-Publication Data

 A catalogue record for this book is available from the National Library of Australia

---

Content Strategist: Melinda McEvoy
Content Project Manager: Shubham Dixit
Edited by Jo Crichton
Proofread by Tim Learner
Copyrights Coordinator: Gobinaath Palanisamy
Cover Designer: Gopalakrishnan Venkatraman
Typeset by Aptara
Printed in China by 1010 Printing International Ltd

Last digit is the print number: 9 8 7 6 5 4 3 2 1

Contents

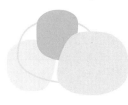# About the author

Gjyn O'Toole has worked in Occupational Therapy, an important health profession for over 40 years. During that time she has provided care for Person/s of all ages, from a diverse number of cultures with various clinical needs, including Team Leadership in Aged Care, and care in Paediatrics, General Rehabilitation, Community Care, Burns, Stroke, Mental Health and Health & Wellbeing education to various age groups. She has also taught as a senior lecturer in various health programs at the University of Newcastle, Australia, for over 20 years.

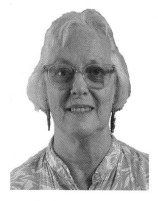

She considers communication to be an essential and foundational skill for achieving effective and appropriate care and thus outcomes within healthcare. Gjyn also acknowledges the importance of Person/Family-centred Care when providing healthcare. She has researched and written a book focusing on communication in healthcare along with other articles and book chapters highlighting aspects of culturally responsive communication, the importance of considering the spiritual aspect of the Person in healthcare and analysis of everyday occupations and life activities. She has taught and lived in various countries including China, Iran and South Africa. Gjyn has also presented her research at conferences relating to health and education in Australia, Africa and Europe.

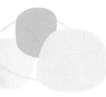

About the resource

Overview

This book has 12 chapters exploring typical aspects of communication in healthcare. These aspects do not cover all relevant aspects; however, in this book they include:

* effective introductions
* gathering information to inform decisions about relevant healthcare, often resulting in comforting or confronting the Person to achieve positive outcomes
* ensuring effective conclusions or closure of interactions or services
* the use of reflection to improve communication
* the use of exploration of personal assumptions and their effect on communication
* the importance of non-verbal aspects of communication
* the relevance of effective listening to inform appropriate healthcare
* the importance of considering the effects of different environments, particularly cultural ones
* the effects of considering the whole person when communicating in healthcare
* effectively managing misunderstandings and possible conflict
* the effective use of telehealth
* the need to consider the responsibility of a healthcare professional when communicating on social media.

These chapters, while exploring each aspect of communication, outline the particular stories of the Person/s receiving healthcare. The focus of the particular chapter provides examples of how a healthcare professional would execute the particular aspect of communication given the particular story of the Person. These interaction examples present stories typical of Person/s with differing needs and backgrounds. These chapters are designed to assist the reader to develop their skills in communication while providing healthcare. It provides a method of exploring and developing relevant communication skills when preparing to become an effective healthcare communicator.

Using this resource

This book is designed to assist individuals to develop effective skills in communication for provision of healthcare. These individuals would typically be undertaking studies to qualify them as a healthcare professional or an assistant healthcare professional. This resource provides opportunities to explore and develop skills in effective communication for those individuals studying any role in healthcare.

The book can be beneficial as a teaching resource to increase awareness of the need for communication skills as well as actual development of those skills while providing healthcare. It can be used in tertiary programs as a self-directed method for developing that awareness and the required skills in communicating during healthcare interactions.

This book can be used online to enable the reader to observe and evaluate the effectiveness of the interactions in the relevant videos, while also considering how to adjust these interactions to achieve more effective communication and satisfying interactions. This has the potential to encourage the development and use of effective communication skills.

While the content of the interactions can be found in the transcripts in the hardcopy of the book, observing the interactions will more effectively inform the reader about the relevant aspect of communication.

Structure of the resource

Stories can be an effective method of learning. Connecting these stories to the reality of the life of the Person has the potential to improve understanding and retention of this understanding about effective communication. It enables the reader to connect aspects of communication to the reality of healthcare communication and the role of the healthcare professional when communicating. This understanding and connection can increase the likelihood of the reader effectively developing their own communication skills. This can promote reflection, thereby enhancing their learning.

As mentioned above, each chapter focuses on an aspect of communication. Within each chapter the provided heading guides the reader to explore and develop an understanding of the focus of the chapter.

REFLECTION

These questions encourage the reader to explore the content of the video and the chapter and then reflect about the content. The questions encourage and potentially guide reflective thinking.

INQUIRY

These questions encourage the reader to explore the effectiveness of this aspect of communication and possible ways to improve the aspect focused upon in the interaction to effectively achieve this aspect of communication.

ACTION

These questions encourage the reader to apply their knowledge and understanding of the particular aspect of communication during all interactions when providing healthcare.

ADDITIONAL ACTIVITIES

These activities are designed to provide an opportunity to explore resources relating to the relevant aspect of effective communication. They also provide ways of practising and evaluating communication skills to enhance these skills during practice.

Acknowledgements

The content of this book results from the many Person/s – women, men, children, families, students and colleagues – with whom I have collaborated over the years to ensure ongoing functioning, health and wellbeing in their everyday life. The combination of these many interactions and collaborative relationships have contributed to the stories of each chapter in this book.

CHAPTER 1

Introductions and providing initial information

INTRODUCTION

Introductions are a part of everyday life, potentially having both positive and negative results. There-fore, considering aspects of effective introductions is essential for the provision of effective healthcare. Successful introductions can result in achieving all aspects of Person/Family-centred Care along with appropriate and reliable interventions.

Person/Family-centred Care requires mutual understanding. This comprises demonstrations of respect, empathy and trustworthiness. It also requires development of a positive therapeutic relationship. Such a relationship requires rapport from a genuine positive connection, effective listening and collaboration. In addition, Person/Family-centred Care results in positive emotions, empowerment of the Person and therefore positive outcomes affecting their satisfaction, health and wellbeing (see Chapter 2 of *Communication: Core interpersonal skills of healthcare professionals,* 5th ed.). Appropriate introductions are an important aspect of effective communication in health practice for both healthcare professionals and for any of the encountered Persons in everyday practice. They contribute to appropriate interven-tions and thus outcomes.

Therefore, introducing the healthcare professional, their role and thus the focus of and procedures relating to their care, aspects of the service and the environment are essential components of effective communication and, thus, care. This process, in most situations also includes the Person providing information relating to themselves and their needs relevant to the role of the particular healthcare professional. This provision of information is typically facilitated by questioning (see Chapter 2 of this book).

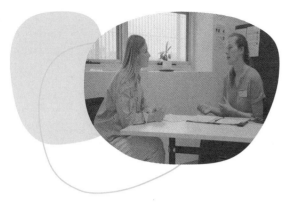

Joan Thomas's story

 View Joan's story or read the transcript.

The Person: Mrs Joan Thomas

In this story, the Person, Mrs Joan Thomas, has been experiencing bilateral knee pain due to osteoarthritis. She has been a ballet dancer for 10 years, resulting in damage to her knees. She is appropriately dressed and, while a little anxious, is happy to be attending a health service to assist with her knee pain. This is especially important to her as she been experiencing increased knee pain recently. She meets the healthcare professional, Meg, for the first time. She hears that this healthcare professional is an Occupational Therapist. She has not heard of that profession. Mrs Joan Thomas and her partner have lived in their current house for 10 years and despite the difficulty of negotiating 15 stairs to enter the house, they do *not* want to move. Mrs Thomas also indicates difficulties with gardening (something she enjoys); getting in and out of bed and using her ensuite toilet comfortably and safely.

The healthcare professional: Meg Smith

The healthcare professional is an Occupational Therapist. She introduces herself using her name, while also exploring with the Person her preferred name. She then explains a few details about the service, providing a print version of these details, while also indicating where to find an appropriate toilet for Mrs Thomas. The explanation results in Meg explaining some aspects of the role of someone in her profession, Occupational Therapy. Following this discussion, Meg confirms factual information about Joan. This leads to realising Joan will be celebrating her birthday in a few days. Meg demonstrates appropriate congratulatory emotions after identifying the approaching birthday. As a result of further discussion, Meg suggests different pieces of assistive aids or equipment to enable Joan to complete her daily tasks more comfortably, including a stair lift; gardening tools; bed raisers to facilitate easy access on and off her bed; a raised toilet seat, along with suggesting a home visit and a referral to a Physiotherapist. During the interaction, Meg demonstrates aspects of Person/Family-centred Care and effective communication.

The setting

Location: A quiet, private room with chairs and a table. The chairs face each other and are a comfortable distance apart.

The context: Outpatient care of the Person (Joan Thomas) with orthopaedic needs. Joan is attending for the first time and is unfamiliar with the health service and the available assistance.

Physical setting: The healthcare professional (Meg Smith) is seated on a chair with a tablet and note pad for recording relevant details of the interaction. The non-verbal messages of Meg indicate complete focus on Joan, thereby demonstrating respect and worthiness of trust.

Reflection

1. What did Meg do to demonstrate respect?
2. If there is anything Meg said that should be different, how would you change it?
3. How did Meg's non-verbal messages affect the interaction?
4. Would the age of the Person affect what you say and how you might say it? If so, how?
5. Consider and describe a time when you felt undervalued because of an ineffective introduction.

Inquiry

1. How effective was this introductory interaction?
2. What did Meg do to develop trust and rapport?
3. How did Meg demonstrate a commitment to Person/Family-centred Care?
4. How did Meg demonstrate effective listening throughout the interaction?

5. How might you change aspects of this interaction to increase effective communication?

Action

1. List the components of an effective introduction.

2. Explain how you would consistently perform effective introductions in practice.

3. Write a description of the role of an Occupational Therapist working with Person/s experiencing orthopaedic conditions.

4. Decide how you would explain your professional role and write a clear concise description of your professional role in either an orthopaedic or an aged-care context.

5. Consider how you might ensure effective introductions in different circumstances; for example, with a semi-conscious Person; with carers or family members and so forth.

Additional activities

1. Refer to Chapter 3 of O'Toole, *Communication: Core interpersonal skills for healthcare professionals*, 5th ed. Choose a scenario from Section 4 and allocate the role of healthcare professional (HcP) and Person. Perform the role play.

2. Reflect on the effectiveness of communication during the role plays to improve performance when interacting in similar circumstances.

   a. Observe and evaluate both the effective and the ineffective aspects of the introduction.

   b. Observe and evaluate demonstration of all aspects of Step 1 of Person/Family-centred Care: Mutual Understanding: Respect, Empathy and Developing Trust.

   c. Observe and evaluate the verbal messages of the healthcare professional.

   d. Observe and evaluate the non-verbal messages of the healthcare professional.

   e. Observe and evaluate the effectiveness of the listening of the healthcare professional.

   f. Consider how your thoughts about introductions have changed and how to apply this.

   g. Suggest how to improve all future introductions in your healthcare profession.

Text link

Chapter 3, 'The specific goals of communication for healthcare professionals: 1 Introductions and providing information'. In O'Toole, G. (2024). *Communication: Core interpersonal skills for healthcare professionals* (5th ed.). Elsevier.

A FINAL WORD

Introductions are foundational in establishing the quality of the therapeutic relationship and the related healthcare. They are reassuring for the Person/s, while also affecting their satisfaction. They ensure effective outcomes for everyone. However, they require the healthcare professional to know the range of care of their employing service. Introductions can be both verbal and written. These forms of introductions must complement each other. Introductions often involve questions to confirm understanding of relevant information and to encourage the often anxious Person/s. Effective introductions should demonstrate all aspects of Person/Family-centred Care and effective communication, thereby preparing the Person/s for future events relating to their care.

Riverdale Inpatient & Community Health Service

Phone: 0456 789 321

This health service provides care for anyone with health needs, whether acute or long term in Orthopaedics; Stroke and General Rehabilitation; Geriatrics and Cardiology.

Healthcare staff

Doctors: We have 4 General Practice doctors (Dr) with different specialties including Orthopaedics; Stroke including General Rehabilitation; Geriatrics; and Cardiology.

Nurses: We have 4 nurses with training and experience in Orthopaedics, Stroke and General Rehabilitation, Aged Care and Cardiology.

Physiotherapists: We have 4 Physiotherapists (PT) who focus on developing movement and muscle strength in any parts of the body to allow their Person/s to life their lives safely and well.

Occupational Therapists: We have 3 Occupational Therapists with training and experience in all the above areas.

Speech Pathologists: We have a Speech Pathologist who focuses on effective communication regardless of the condition.

Social Workers: We have a Social Worker who can assist in exploring appropriate places for you to live and to explore providing you with appropriate services in your home.

The role of the Occupational Therapist

Occupational Therapists focus on the activities you do every day. They seek to help you to complete these activities safely and independently during your daily life. They consider the difficulties you have completing your required and desired activities because of your condition.

This means they consider your difficulties while showering or bathing; going to the toilet; getting dressed and undressed; getting in and out of bed; sitting in and getting out of your lounge chairs and/or dining chairs; making meals, hot drinks, or snacks; shopping; driving; gardening or any other things you enjoy doing that may not be absolutely necessary to your life but provide enjoyment for you (they call them leisure activities); being able to use stairs; and doing challenging work activities (they call it Work Health Safety activities). They also work with people with mental health difficulties to enable them to do all their daily activities.

In order to assist you with some of these activities, they can come to your home to assess and suggest pieces of equipment to assist you to do particular activities safely and independently. They can also make suggestions of how to modify aspects of your home to make it safer; for example, installing a rail or ramp or stair lift to help you to be safe and independent. These can help you to avoid falls and any other possible injuries.

If you have any questions about this service and the staff, please ask at the desk.

CHAPTER 2

Questioning, leading to comforting and confronting

INTRODUCTION

Questions are a common aspect of communication in daily life. They are helpful in learning about those around us. However, in the provision of healthcare, they are essential aspects of effective communication. The answers to questions have the potential to provide appropriate information for development of relevant and effective interventions. The importance of answers to questions in this context indicate the need to use questions and particular types of questions appropriately. Such answers not only provide relevant information for the healthcare professional, but they also provide information to facilitate relevant comfort for and sometimes appropriate confrontation of the Person/s relating to their needs.

There are two major types of questions. A closed question (these include multiple-choice questions where the individual asking the question provides several options as possible answers) seeks a short and specific answer – sometimes yes or no and other times a simple word or two, thereby providing the required information. The other type of questions, open questions, allows for 'open' answers. These answers provide more detailed information about various aspects of the needs of the Person/s. They may take some time for the Person/s to answer, while expressing ideas in many sentences.

Answers to questions also provide the opportunity to respectfully relate to the Person/s. Answers to questions often express distressing or difficult emotions, thereby allowing the healthcare professional to comfort the Person/s. Expression of emotions may also identify the need to respectfully challenge the emotions or habits of the Person/s, especially when relating to their future improvement.

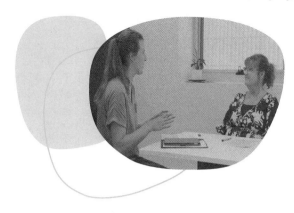

Mrs Richards' story

View Mrs Richards' story or read the transcript.

The Person: Mrs Richards

In this story, Mrs Richards has injured her right shoulder, affecting the use of her arm and her hand. This is her dominant side and thus has major effects on her everyday life. These effects include showering and dressing; making a hot drink; driving and other activities relevant to her daily life. She had not been to this health service for over a year, prior to coming in last week. During that time a variety of things have changed requiring clarifying and sometimes updating records. This is not the first time Mrs Richards has seen this healthcare professional, Meg Smith, and thus she appears relatively relaxed. However, she has a few questions relating to her treatment. These questions indicate her desire to have definitive answers, aligning with her own preferences. Despite her commitment to ongoing treatment, she would like to finish as soon as possible and, in order to avoid disappointment, without establishing some goals. Due to other commitments in her life, she is not always able to complete her recommended exercises, which are necessary for her improvement. This could lengthen her need for ongoing treatment. While she understands this, the fatigue she experiences overcomes her need to complete the relevant exercises.

The healthcare professional: Meg Smith

The healthcare professional must confirm the details of each particular Person, including contact details, such as their address and phone numbers. The healthcare professional therefore asks questions to gather information and sometimes to clarify this gathered information. In this story, Meg asks Mrs Richards to confirm her address and her phone numbers. However, before confirming these details, she begins the interaction with a question relating to her previous session with Mrs Richards. This question ensures the satisfaction of Mrs Richards, potentially reducing any anxiety or negative feelings. Sometimes, family members of the Person may have questions relating to the ongoing healthcare of the Person, thereby making the initial question important.

After confirming the address and phone numbers for Mrs Richards, Meg then asks about her listed conditions. This identifies a condition previously not recorded in the medical records. The identified condition could have substantial effects on the progress of Mrs Richards and the expectations of Meg. Meg also asks about the current pain levels of Mrs Richards to assist in confirming if there has been improvement. After updating the medical records, Meg focuses on the current reasons for this session – the injured right shoulder, which is the dominant arm of Mrs Richards. The interaction also identifies that Mrs Richards does not like to set goals. During the following interaction, Mrs Richards tells Meg she is going away with her husband. This results in further questions to ensure safety and success during the trip, as Mrs Richards cannot attend the following weekly session. Meg asks questions relating to the commitment of Mrs Richards to completing her suggested exercises throughout the day. Responding to these questions is not only confronting for Mrs Richards but also comforting as she is acknowledged for the daily challenges she experiences.

The questions assist in the provision of important information relevant to the care of Mrs Richards. The answers to these questions potentially reduce the time spent on finding them if necessary, thereby reducing wasted time for Meg. They can also lead to both comfort and confrontation during practice. Both of these can be essential in satisfying and having a positive outcome for the Person/s and the healthcare professional.

The setting

Location: A quiet, private space in an outpatient treatment area, with the Person (Mrs Richards) seated and facing the healthcare professional (Meg Smith) a comfortable distance away.

The context: An outpatient setting in a private space, with the healthcare professional meeting the Person to gather information relevant to the needs of the Person and the profession of the healthcare professional. Gathering this information assists in the provision of relevant interventions and ongoing care. Mrs Richards is receiving treatment for an injured right (R) shoulder.

Physical setting: Mrs Richards and Meg are sitting a comfortable distance apart, opposite each other (facing each other), one on the end of the table and the other on the closest side of the table. Meg has either a notebook or a computer/tablet for recording answers to her questions.

Reflection

1. Identify the questions potentially developing rapport and state how they might develop rapport (a therapeutic relationship).

2. Identify those questions indicating understanding of the reality of life for Mrs Richards and state what aspects of Person/Family-centred Care they could develop.

3. Identify the closed questions and what they achieved.

4. Consider the use of non-verbal communication when asking questions and decide how to ensure you always use appropriate non-verbal communication when asking questions,
   a. when comforting, and
   b. when confronting.

5. If watching the video, how did Meg's non-verbal cues demonstrate all aspects of Person/Family-centred Care and effective communication?

Inquiry

1. How effective were Meg's questions in gathering relevant information and why?

2. Why did Mrs Richards' closed questions not always achieve a desired short answer?

3. How effective were Meg's responses in demonstrating comfort? Explain why.

4. a. How and why were the questions relating to confronting the need to exercise four times a day relevant to Mrs Richards and her needs?
   b. What might such questions and confrontation achieve for Mrs Richards?

Action

1. State the types of questions, and write several examples of each type of question, relevant to your healthcare profession.

2. Consider situations in healthcare requiring comfort and create questions relevant to those situations.

3. Suggest possible circumstances requiring confrontation when working as a healthcare professional and indicate questions relevant to managing such circumstances.

4. When providing healthcare, are there any other people who the healthcare professional might need to question, comfort and/or confront? Who are they and how will you ensure effective questioning and therefore effective outcomes?

Additional activities

Refer to Chapter 4 of O'Toole, *Communication: Core interpersonal skills for healthcare professionals*, 5th ed., to complete the following.

1. Mrs Richards asks three closed questions (she is seeking a definite answer) – however, the answers are not always a simple closed question answer.
   a. Consider and list other situations when the answer to a closed question provides more than a simple, one-point answer.
   b. Decide how you might manage such situations in healthcare.

2. a. Identify the closed questions and what they achieved for Meg.
   b. What did they achieve for Mrs Richards?

3. a. Identify the open questions and what they achieved for Meg.
   b. What did they achieve for Mrs Richards?

Text link

Chapter 4, 'The specific goals of communication for healthcare professionals: 2 Questioning, comforting and confronting. In O'Toole, G. (2024). *Communication: Core interpersonal skills for healthcare professionals* (5th ed.). Elsevier.

A FINAL WORD

Questions are an essential aspect of effective communication and thus healthcare, they can gather information, clarify understanding and probe to gather necessary information. They affect not only the quality of the relationship with the Person, they also contribute substantially to the quality of care for the Person. They include questions designed to gather simple one-point answers and those designed to gather more information relevant to the Person, their needs and the particular healthcare profession. Questions can result in comforting the Person and often confronting them in order to ensure satisfactory outcomes. These aspects of communication therefore contribute to the achievement of Person/Family-centred Care for all Persons, thereby achieving effective communication and outcomes for those involved in that care.

CHAPTER 3
Effective closure of interactions and services

INTRODUCTION

Closure or conclusions of inpatient or outpatient services in healthcare are a reality. They are often considered a normal procedure for the healthcare professional, although not necessarily for the Person/s. Effective closure, whether for a single session or interaction, or for a period of regular care, or closure due to a palliative condition, reflects upon the healthcare professional and their service. Effective closures require planning and recognition of the approaching conclusion of care. This involves awareness of the length of individual sessions, the possible timeframe for achievement of established goals (often established by the healthcare professional after assessment of and discussion with the Person/s), along with the expected improvement of their condition given the particular needs and/or circumstances of each Person/s. Effective closures require mutual understanding of the purpose of sessions and the expectations for improvement and conclusion of services. They also require a summary of achievements and clarification of understanding of these achievements for both the Person/s and the healthcare professional. Effective closure ensures satisfaction and appropriate outcomes for both the Person and the healthcare professional.

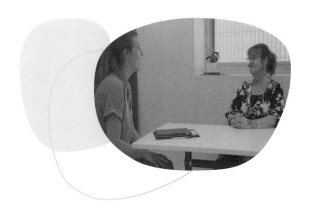

Mrs Richards' story

 View Mrs Richards' story or read the transcript.

The Person: Mrs Richards

In this story, the Person, Mrs Richards, has injured her right shoulder, affecting the use of her hand. She has been attending the service for several months.

Mrs Richards has seen the same healthcare professional, Meg Smith, for one-hourly sessions each week. She has also seen other healthcare professionals relevant to her needs. Her mood, initially depressed and unmotivated, has become more interested and engaged in her treatment, but also the expectations of her daily life. In addition, Mrs Richards is more able to use her right arm and hand, regularly doing more with them. Despite her improvement, she is still a little reluctant and anxious. She has, however, developed the ability to open doors, unbutton and take off her jacket and complete all expectations at work, although a little more slowly than previously, along with controlling her strong emotional outbursts. Mrs Richards would like to be able to drive again, despite her partner enjoying driving her to and from work. It provides time alone without the demanding children.

Mrs Richards enjoys attending the clinic for treatment and does not respond well to the reminder that it finishes in two weeks. She is not sure her improvement has been as positive as suggested, indicating her reluctance to stop attending.

The healthcare professional: Meg Smith

The healthcare professional, Meg Smith, has been seeing the Person, Mrs Richards, for several months. During this time she has been able to assist Mrs Richards in improving both her emotional control and her use of her right arm and hand. Meg is preparing to conclude the 10 weeks of intervention and thus discusses this with Mrs Richards. She intends to assist Mrs Richards to prepare for the closure of their sessions by mentioning that this will occur in two weeks. She reassures Mrs Richards, identifying her level of improvement in the activities of her daily life, in her work and in her emotional control and her sleep habits. Meg also indicates her satisfaction with this improvement, and articulates her understanding and thankfulness for Mrs Richards regularly following the exercise guidelines provided by another healthcare professional.

Meg learns about the benefit of Mrs Richards being driven to work by her partner. She also acknowledges the concern of Mrs Richards about concluding her treatment. She reinforces the improvement of Mrs Richards and her achievement of the goals discussed in the first session. Meg indicates her enjoyment of regularly meeting with Mrs Richards, reminding her that Mrs Richards can contact Meg if she feels the need to talk. When concluding any sessions, whether or not multiple, it can be important to ensure the Person/s has relevant contact details to answer any questions and to ensure ongoing improvement and satisfaction.

The setting

Location: A quiet private space with chairs and a table. The chairs face each other, one at the end of the table and the other facing the other chair alongside the table.

The context: This is an outpatient service. The Person, Mrs Richards, has been attending this service for one-hour sessions for eight consecutive weeks. She has been seeing the same healthcare professional, Meg Smith, during this time. She has also seen other healthcare professionals relevant to her needs.

Physical setting: Meg and Mrs Richards are seated opposite each other. Meg has a device next to her on the table. She often refers to this device to confirm particular details.

The healthcare professional, Meg, is looking at her device checking Mrs Richards' records relating to the expected duration of overall treatment and the goals established in week 1 for Mrs Richards. She also confirms her memory that Mrs Richards, at the beginning of treatment, was told to expect 10 weeks of treatment.

Reflection

1. What did Meg do to demonstrate the need for a respectful conclusion to the existing therapeutic relationship?

2. If watching the video, what were the effects of Meg's non-verbal messages on the interaction?

3. How did Meg demonstrate aspects of Person/Family-centred Care, empowering Mrs Richards for her future?

4. How might you ensure effective closure of multiple sessions for the healthcare professional and the Person?

5. Consider and describe a time when you felt undervalued because of an ineffective conclusion to an interaction or multiple planned events.

Inquiry

1. How effective was this discussion for concluding this session?

2. How effective was the discussion for preparation of the conclusion of the 10 weeks of treatment?

3. What did Meg do to summarise previous discussions and thus clarify understanding?

4. How did Meg demonstrate a commitment to Person/Family-centred Care?

5. Using effective communication, how might you change aspects of this interaction to achieve a satisfying and effective conclusion?

Action

1. List the components of effective conclusions when offering relevant healthcare.

2. Explain how you would consistently perform effective conclusions in practice.

3. List the possible effects of inappropriate conclusions to healthcare for the Person.

4. List the possible effects of inappropriate conclusions to healthcare for the healthcare professional.

5. Describe how you might ensure effective conclusions in different contexts; for example, if working in inpatient care; or with carers or family members; or in outpatient care; or in the home of the Person; or with children and so forth.

Additional activities

1. Refer to Chapter 5 of O'Toole, *Communication: Core interpersonal skills for healthcare professionals*, 5th ed. Choose a scenario from Section 4 and allocate the role of healthcare professional and Person. Perform the role play.

2. Reflect on the effectiveness of communication during the role plays to improve performance when interacting in similar circumstances.

   a. Observe and evaluate both the effective and the ineffective aspects of the conclusion.

   b. Observe and evaluate demonstration of all aspects of Step 1 of Person/Family-centred Care: Mutual Understanding: Respect, Empathy and Developing Trust.

   c. Observe and evaluate the verbal messages of the healthcare professional.

   d. Observe and evaluate the non-verbal messages of the healthcare professional.

   e. Observe and evaluate the effectiveness of the listening of the healthcare professional.

   f. Consider how your thoughts about conclusions have changed and how to apply this.

   g. Suggest how to improve all future conclusions of treatment in your healthcare profession.

Text link

Chapter 5, 'The specific goals of communication for healthcare professionals: 3 Effective conclusions of interactions and services: Negotiating closure. In O'Toole, G. (2024). *Communication: Core interpersonal skills for healthcare professionals* (5th ed.). Elsevier.

A FINAL WORD

Closures or conclusions are important in confirming the quality of the related healthcare and the therapeutic relationship. They are reassuring and satisfying for the Person/s, while also confirming the interest and commitment of the healthcare professional in empowering the Person. Thus, they ensure effective outcomes for everyone. However, they require the healthcare professional to consider the features of an effective and satisfying conclusion. Closures, in common with all communication, involve both verbal and non-verbal messages. These aspects of communication must complement each other to ensure mutual understanding. Conclusions often involve questions to confirm understanding of relevant information and to encourage the often anxious Person/s. They can also involve summaries of the content of both immediate and previous sessions. Effective closure demonstrates all aspects of effective communication and Person/Family-centred Care, thereby preparing the Person/s for their future without healthcare.

CHAPTER 4

Reflective practice

INTRODUCTION

Reflection is an important element of practice. It is sometimes avoided due to time constraints or reluctance on the part of the healthcare professional. However, it contributes to effective communication by facilitating understanding of responses during all interactions while providing healthcare. These interactions can occur with fellow healthcare service employees (including students, cleaners and maintenance staff); individual Persons, along with their carers or family members, and any other individuals regularly relating to the individual Person; for example, teachers or homecare nurses. Reflection also enables the healthcare professional to be aware of the causes of their personal reactions during interactions, thereby promoting effective communication. It can develop understanding of the effects of personality and related communication styles upon interactions and relationships. This can assist in accommodating these aspects of self thereby encouraging demonstration of Person/Family-centred Care in healthcare.

Exploring Reflection PowerPoint slides

 Watch the PowerPoint presentation video.

The content of the PowerPoint slides is listed below, however it does not include the discussion relevant to each slide, which you will find in the video.

Slide 1 Introductory: EXPLORING REFLECTION: Achieving effective communication in healthcare through reflection

Slide 2 Reflection about communicative interactions

- is a conscious exploration of interactions
- may occur during an interaction or after the interaction
- allows the healthcare professional (HcP) to understand

- enables changes to ensure the development of effective communication.

Slide 3 Reflection achieves learning and possible growth

- Facilitates learning about yourself
- Learning about your colleagues
- Learning about the Person/s you assist or enable
- Can facilitate learning about service policies and guidelines

Slide 4 REFLECTION

- is not natural to all personality types
- may require commitment
- may initially require dedicated time to develop skills in reflection
- may initially require a model of reflection to develop those skills.

Slide 5 Possible Models of Reflection

Models of Reflection can guide the reflective process.

- ✔ Kolb – a learning cycle (1984)
- ✔ Boud, Keogh & Walker (1985)

✔ Gibbs (1988)

✔ Fish, Twinn & Purr (1991)

✔ Johns (2022)

✔ O'Toole (2024)

Slide 6 A healthcare-related model to guide reflective care

Step 1 Choosing to and allocating time to Reflect about your healthcare practice.

Step 2 Choose a Challenging or Interesting Event.

Step 3 Describe and Explore the Chosen Event.

Step 4 Explore ALL reactions: Self and the Person/s.

Step 5 Establish relevant Goals for similar future events or interactions.

Step 6 Develop strategies and/or Future Action Plans.

Step 7 Act to Fulfil the Plans: Reflecting upon and Changing Healthcare, as necessary.

(O'Toole 2024, p. 79)

Slide 7 Using Reflection in practice can increase:

- self and Person/s awareness
- awareness of areas of strength
- awareness of areas for improvement
- understanding and honesty
- predictability
- competence in communication and practice.

Slide 8 References (see page 42)

Text links

Chapter 6, 'Awareness of and the need for reflective practice in healthcare communication' and Chapter 7, 'Awareness of self to enhance healthcare communication'. In O'Toole, G. (2024). *Communication: Core interpersonal skills for healthcare professionals* (5th ed.). Elsevier.

Reflection

1. What have you learnt about reflection today?

2. How might reflection assist in identifying your strengths and areas for improvement?

3. How might reflection empower you to use your strengths to develop in areas requiring improvement?

4. How might the steps in the model on Slide 6 assist you to develop skills in reflection?

5. How might reflection assist in achieving Person/Family-centred Care?

Inquiry

1. Do you agree that reflection has positive effects for the healthcare professional? If so, why? If not, why not?

2. How might reflection benefit the Person/s the healthcare professional is assisting?

3. Why do you think a model of reflection might assist the reflection process, even for individuals who have reflective personalities?

4. Do you feel the steps of the model on Slide 6 would suit you to enable reflection? If so, why? If not, why not?

5. How might reflection achieve the listed benefits on slide 7?

Action

Explain how you would consistently use reflection in practice.

1. Choose a positive interaction and isolate what you did to make it positive.

2. Choose an unsatisfactory interaction, use the steps of the model of reflection to identify the causes relevant to you and establish an action plan for future similar interactions.

3. Use the answers to 2 and 3 to identify your strengths.

4. Establish how you will ensure use of your strengths to develop areas for improvement to consistently develop effective communication skills in healthcare.

Additional activities

Refer to Chapters 6 and 7 of O'Toole, *Communication: Core interpersonal skills for healthcare professionals*, 5th ed., in combination with the PowerPoint slides, to complete the following in groups or pairs.

1. State the relevance of reflection to daily healthcare.

2. Explore and decide how reflection and awareness of self can benefit all interactions, within and outside the provision of healthcare.

3. List and discuss the benefits of identifying your strengths and areas requiring improvement for both your professional and your personal life.

4. State the advantage of knowing your strengths for interactions in healthcare.

5. Decide how to use your strengths to improve and potentially overcome your areas for improvement.

A FINAL WORD

Reflection in healthcare practice has the potential for increasing the quality of interactions, thereby achieving effective communication. It facilitates learning about self (self-awareness) and about others, typically the Person/s and health professional colleagues, along with policies and guidelines relevant to healthcare. Reflection requires commitment and allocation of dedicated time, whether daily or weekly. Developing skills in reflection may benefit from the use of a relevant model of reflection. There are a variety available, however the O'Toole model is relevant to the healthcare context. It has seven steps designed to facilitate understanding of self and others while also developing action plans to ensure effective communication and Person/Family-centred interactions and, thus, the quality of care.

CHAPTER 5

Personal assumptions affecting communication

INTRODUCTION

Personal assumptions (also known as stereotyping) about others are typically used at the beginning of interactions. They can be based on the appearance of an individual; for example, how they are dressed, their jewellery or tattoos; or a particular behaviour; for example, always arriving late or smoking; or the job they have – for example, a cleaner, a corporate manager or a truck driver; and sometimes on the tone of voice and associated actions. Assumptions, however, do not always create an appropriate understanding of the other individual. A healthcare professional assuming particular things about Person/s (potentially stereotyping them) has the potential to negatively affect interactions with the Person/s. These can produce ongoing challenges when interacting with the Person/s. Such assumptions can also result in misunderstandings and often incorrect information, producing inappropriate care. These affect the possibility of demonstrating all elements of Person/Family-centred Care, indicating the need for a healthcare professional to always relate to those around them with positive attitudes without assumption, prejudice or stereotyping.

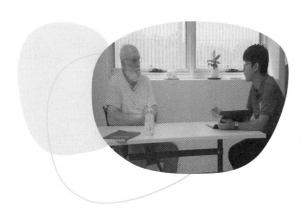

Frank's story

> View Frank's story or read the transcript.

The Person: Mr Frank Bennet

In this story, the Person, Frank, attends a health service for the first time, because of an injured dominant left hand. On this occasion, he is dressed in ragged and obviously grubby clothing. He is quite forceful and obviously unhappy. While Frank appears determined, he also seems flustered and stressed. Upon seeing the healthcare professional, Michael, they speak loudly and inappropriately about the possible age and competence of Michael. Frank is not happy to learn this healthcare professional is the one he will be seeing. He does not respond well to Michael or to his assumptions about Frank.

When a friend, Alex, another healthcare professional, comes to see him during the session with Michael, Frank relaxes, indicating pleasure at the arrival of Alex. He interacts with Alex indicating pleasure, while admitting his family made this appointment for him and for an assessment of his dominant left hand.

The healthcare professional 1: Michael Wang

This healthcare professional, Michael, has been working at this service for five years, despite appearing the age of a school student. He explains this to the Person, Frank, while also suggesting he could see a different healthcare professional if he was willing to wait for possibly more than an hour for this. He has assumed Frank does not take adequate care of himself because of his appearance and, according to the referral, he has injured his left hand. Michael automatically assumes Frank has not injured his dominant hand, as most people are right-handed.

Michael is relieved when a different healthcare professional from the service, Alex, comes to see Frank. Michael listens to the conversation, admitting the error of his assumption about the dominant hand of Frank. As a result of the conversation between Frank and Alex, Michael begins the interaction with Frank again with a completely different attitude. He apologises for his assumptions and begins the interaction with a more positive attitude. This different attitude allows Michael to identify why Frank was so stressed when arriving at the service.

The healthcare professional 2: Alex Jones

This healthcare professional, Alex, is a friend of Frank and upon learning he had an appointment today, Alex told Michael he would come to briefly see Frank. His knowledge and conversation with Frank identifies the reason for his appearance, while also highlighting that the injury was to his dominant hand, despite it being the left hand.

The setting

Location: Initially in a waiting area of an outpatient health service. Then moving to a quiet private room with chairs and a table in the room. Michael and Frank sit a comfortable distance from each other, while also facing each other.

The context: An outpatient service, initially a waiting area and then a private space. Frank is attending for the first time.

Physical setting: Initially, the waiting room of an outpatient service and then a quiet space.

Reflection

1. What do you usually base your ideas (assumptions or judgments) about a Person on?

2. Have these assumptions caused misunderstandings in the past? How have you overcome them?

3. What stereotypical judgments do you typically make about other people?

4. How do you overcome the tendency to make assumptions or stereotype people you do not know, who are different to you?

5. How do you feel when others make assumptions about you or stereotype you, whether or not they are accurate?

Inquiry

1. How did Frank's assumptions affect the interaction?

2. How did Michael's assumptions affect the interaction?

3. What caused the interaction to improve for Frank?

4. What enabled Michael to overcome his assumptions about Frank?

5. How might you change aspects of this interaction to avoid making assumptions and stereotypical judgments?

Action

1. List the possible ways to overcome personal assumptions and the tendency to stereotype others.

2. Consider and identify how you would consistently avoid making assumptions in practice.

3. Decide how you would respond when others make assumptions about you, in practice, that are hurtful or produce pain for you.

4. Suggest how to overcome the effects of someone assuming things about you or stereotyping you in practice.

5. Consider how making assumptions and stereotypes might affect the achievement of effective communication and Person/Family-centred Care.

Additional activities

Refer to Chapters 6, 7 and 8 of O'Toole, *Communication: Core interpersonal skills for healthcare professionals*, 5th ed, to complete the following in groups or pairs.

1. Suggest how to ensure achievement of effective communication when experiencing assumptions or stereotyping.

2. Suggest how to maintain unconditional positive regard for those who make negative assumptions about you in practice.

3. Suggest how to ensure consistent unconditional positive regard for Person/s in practice who have a lifestyle you find difficult to accept or a life situation you feel is inappropriate but a result of their own decisions and behaviour.

4. Suggest how to continue aiming to consistently achieve all aspects of the first step of Person/Family-centred Care – Mutual Understanding, when experiencing negative personal assumptions and/or stereotyping in practice.

5. Suggest how to develop rapport and listen actively when the Person is assuming things about you or stereotyping you inappropriately.

Text links

Chapter 6, 'Awareness of and the need for reflective practice in healthcare communication'; Chapter 7, 'Awareness of self to enhance healthcare communication' and Chapter 8, 'Awareness of how personal assumptions affect healthcare communication'. In O'Toole, G. (2024). Communication: Core interpersonal skills for healthcare professionals (5th ed.). Elsevier.

A FINAL WORD

Personal assumptions are a reality in life. However, they do not always have positive results. They are typically based on the beliefs and values of the individual making the assumptions. These tendencies are best avoided when practising as a healthcare professional. They have the potential to produce not only uncomfortable interactions, but also a negative reputation for the assuming healthcare professional. Any Person requiring assistance from a healthcare professional will feel vulnerable. These feelings of vulnerability may produce strong negative emotions and application of assumptions about the healthcare professional. It is essential for all healthcare professionals to avoid responding negatively to such assumptions as well as avoiding making assumptions themselves. Practising without making assumptions or stereotyping has the potential to produce not only Person/Family-centred care, but also effective communication and, thus, quality healthcare.

Non-verbal communication

INTRODUCTION

Non-verbal communication is always present in every interaction. It affects all interactions, carrying sometimes over 80 per cent of a message. It can also change the meaning of the words, depending on various aspects of non-verbal messages. It not only complements the spoken words, but it also emphasises and clarifies the intended meaning. It certainly affects the types of emotions occurring during an interaction. It can improve the mood or create negative feelings during an interaction. Non-verbal messages consist of facial expressions, gestures, body position, eye contact, and expression through the voice, including tone, pitch, speed, pauses, laughing, groaning and so forth, along with the use of pauses and a time of silence within an interaction and sometimes the distance between the interacting individuals. Non-verbal communication indicates the focus and interest of the healthcare professional throughout the interaction. In order to achieve effective communication, it is essential that the words and non-verbal messages combine to send the same message. This will improve the quality of the interaction along with the satisfaction of all participants.

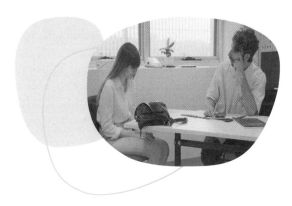

Toni's story

 View Toni's story or read the transcript.

The Person: Toni

In this story, the Person, Toni, lives alone. She has been seeing this healthcare professional, Glen, for several months for management of back pain. Her pet bird died recently. This bird spoke to her multiple times each day and was an enjoyable and constant companion. Unfortunately, her one remaining companion, her dog, is now ill. The vet is concerned about the dog, due to its age and the severity of the illness. The vet has indicated they will do everything they can to keep the dog alive; however, taking the dog for daily hour-long walks along the seashore (a regular enjoyable activity for Toni and the dog) will not be possible anymore. During the discussion of these details, Toni must wonder whether or not Glen is actually listening due to his non-verbal messages.

Toni is obviously upset, crying at any mention of the bird or dog. She had intended to give the toys and cage belonging to the bird to some children who loved birds. When Glen mentions this, she sobs while non-verbally indicating she wants Glen to stop talking. When Glen firmly asks about completing daily exercises to improve her function and reduce her pain, Toni begins crying again. She has been so distressed that she has not been able to do anything in the past few weeks. She actually cannot even remember what she was supposed to do. When Glen leaves the room to collect a printed copy of the exercises and precautions, Toni relaxes a little. As some time passes and she needs to go to the toilet, she stands and moves towards the door.

The healthcare professional: Glen Collins

The healthcare professional, Glen, is obviously distracted and focusing on other aspects of his life. He repeatedly looks at his mobile phone and even sometimes appears to be sending messages using the phone. He hears some of the content of the verbal messages of Toni, especially after noticing her obvious distress. When Toni begins sobbing, Glen stops focusing on his mobile phone and moves towards Toni in order to comfort her. Before touching Toni, Glen asks if he can place his arm around her shoulder. Glen sits quietly with his arm around her shoulder, waiting for her to relax. He does, however, continue looking at his mobile phone.

When Toni indicates non-verbally that she is feeling better, Glen suggests the experience of losing two valued pet companions would be very difficult. Having acknowledged these feelings, Glen then asks if Toni has been completing the previously discussed activities and exercises. Upon hearing a 'no' answer, he states that her health and self-care is important and needs to be a priority, stressing the necessity of completing those activities and exercises. Glen identifies that Toni cannot really remember their previous discussion about activities and exercises. Glen offers to print a copy of these so Toni can read them when she feels better. This takes more time than expected. When he returns to the room with the printout Glen responds quite strongly to Toni who is about to leave the room. He is not happy when Toni indicates he has been gone more than five minutes and she needs to go to the toilet. With some frustration and impatience in his voice Glen confirms that Toni knows where to find the toilet.

The setting

Location: A quiet room in an outpatient service with a table and chairs facing each other a comfortable distance apart.

The context: The Person (Toni) has been seeing this healthcare professional, Glen Collins, regularly, every fortnight for several months. They are familiar with each other and thus are usually relaxed and happy when interacting. Today there is negative emotion due to the recent loss of a valued pet and now the possible loss of the one remaining pet that provides company for Toni who lives alone.

Physical setting: Glen has a mobile phone and a tablet for note taking. Toni and Glen are sitting opposite each other at a table.

Reflection

1. If any of the non-verbal messages of the healthcare professional should be different, how would you change them?
2. What non-verbal messages did Glen use to demonstrate empathy?
3. How do you typically use non-verbal cues when interacting with others?
4. How might you adjust your non-verbal messages when interacting as a healthcare professional?
5. List particular non-verbal messages that demonstrate effective and active listening.

Inquiry

1. How did the non-verbal messages of Glen affect the interaction?
2. What were the different non-verbal messages of Toni and what did they communicate?
3. How did Glen demonstrate a commitment to Person/Family-centred Care?
4. What did the non-verbal messages of Toni communicate?
5. How might you change aspects of this interaction to achieve effective communication?

Action

1. List all components of non-verbal communication.
2. Explain how you would consistently use each of the non-verbal components in practice.
3. Write a list of those non-verbal messages that contribute to Person/Family-centred Care.
4. Decide how you would consistently use appropriate non-verbal messages in daily practice.
5. Consider how you might ensure effective communication and Person/Family-centred Care using non-verbal messages.

Additional activities

1. Refer to Chapter 10 of O'Toole, *Communication: Core interpersonal skills for healthcare professionals*, 5th ed. Choose a scenario from Section 4 and allocate the role of healthcare professional and Person. Perform the role play.

2. Reflect on the non-verbal aspects of communication during the role plays to improve the appropriate use of non-verbal cues when interacting in practice.

   a. Observe and evaluate both the effective and the ineffective aspects of non-verbal messages.

   b. Observe and evaluate the use of non-verbal cues to demonstrate all aspects of Step 1 of Person/Family-centred Care: Mutual Understanding: Respect, Empathy and Developing Trust.

   c. Observe and evaluate the effect of the non-verbal messages of the healthcare professional on their verbal messages.

   d. Observe and evaluate the effect of the non-verbal messages of the Person on the healthcare professional.

   e. Observe and evaluate the effectiveness of the listening.

   f. Consider how your thoughts about non-verbal messages have changed and how to apply this understanding to interactions with the Person and all colleagues in practice.

   g. Suggest how to improve the use of non-verbal cues for all future interactions.

Text link

Chapter 10, 'Awareness of the effects of non-verbal communication for the healthcare professional'. In O'Toole, G. (2024*). Communication: Core interpersonal skills for healthcare professionals* (5th ed.). Elsevier.

A FINAL WORD

All interactions in healthcare involve the use of non-verbal communication. The non-verbal messages of the Person provide deeper understanding of the emotional state of the Person relating to the management of their condition and their needs. Confirmation of this understanding will assist the healthcare professional to provide effective and quality care. In addition, the non-verbal messages of the healthcare professional must be used carefully to ensure appropriate and effective communication. Although it is understandable that during a busy day the healthcare professional may not always use non-verbal communication appropriately with those around them, it is important that the healthcare professional is always aware of their non-verbal messages, including the tone of their voice, their facial expressions, their body position, along with their appearance, cleanliness, organisation and tidiness. Non-verbal communication contributes substantially to the effectiveness of communication, Person/Family-centred Care and, therefore, the quality of healthcare.

CHAPTER 7

Effective listening to achieve understanding

INTRODUCTION

Effective listening is essential for effective communication in healthcare. It requires a focus on and consideration of the whole Person/s, along with a commitment to achieving mutual understanding. It requires a consistent and conscious focus on the Person/s and the content of the interaction, thereby facilitating appropriate responses to all verbal and non-verbal messages. This focus demonstrates respect, interest and acceptance, contributing to the development of a therapeutic relationship. Effective listening requires preparation, by deliberately reducing distractions and possible interruptions. It is demonstrated through all non-verbal messages, including body position and placement, facial expressions, tone of voice and gestures. It requires understanding of typical listening barriers. These barriers can markedly reduce the effectiveness of listening during any interaction. Effective listening also requires satisfying conclusions to interactions or sessions for the Person/s. It is important for achieving Person/Family-centred Care.

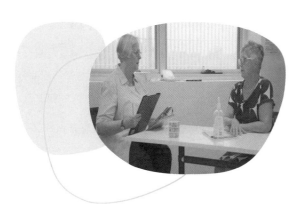

Mrs Stein's story

 View Mrs Stein's story or read the transcript.

The Person: Mrs Stein

In this story, Mrs Stein has been experiencing pain. She lives with her disabled sister and her husband who is not recovering well from a recent fall. She has had three weeks of treatment with the same healthcare professional, Pat. She has currently been sitting in a room for some time, waiting for Pat to arrive. She is beginning to feel impatient and frustrated.

When Pat finally arrives, the initial relief of Mrs Stein, soon turns to frustration again. She finds Pat annoying as she constantly interrupts her, finishing her sentences with incorrect information. Her level of frustration increases a little when Pat asks her for information that should already be in her medical records. However, Mrs Stein complies and provides the information (the number of the homecare service assisting her). Her frustration and impatience increases when Pat responds to a message on her personal mobile phone relating to her plans for the evening.

After repeated interruptions from Pat with incorrect assumptions about Mrs Stein's progress and needing to leave the room to find a required document for her manager, Mrs Stein says Pat should practise *listening*! Listening carefully; avoiding distractions not relevant to Mrs Stein and focusing on her, might assist Pat to remember relevant information about each Person she assists and other requirements of her work. In addition, relevant details about a Person would typically be entered into the relevant medical file, making it even more challenging to understand the various responses of Pat.

Mrs Stein finishes this interaction with the comment: 'Finally you remember something relevant about me!'

The healthcare professional: Pat Bates

Pat appears preoccupied and easily distracted by other aspects of her life. She often looks directly at Mrs Stein, while often responding inappropriately and using her personal mobile phone. She also repeatedly completes the sentences of Mrs Stein with incorrect information. This and the need to leave the room as a result of not listening during a staff meeting the previous day, indicates her lack of skills in effective listening. After finding the relevant document for her manager and returning to the room, she mentions her ineffective listening after a long and busy day yesterday.

The issue Mrs Stein has been experiencing and relevant information about her life, appear to be things Pat either has not remembered or cannot remember due to ineffective listening. During the interaction, Mrs Stein suggests Pat should practise listening. Pat is surprised, saying she thinks she is a good listener!

The setting

Location: A quiet private room with chairs a comfortable distance apart and a table.

The context: An outpatient service which the Person, Mrs Stein, has been attending for ongoing treatment (one-hour sessions) for the previous three weeks, seeing the same healthcare professional.

Physical setting: Initially the healthcare professional, Pat, is outside the room about to enter. Pat enters the room, sitting on a chair facing Mrs Stein.

Reflection

1. What are the possible effects of the listening style of Pat upon the quality of care?
2. What listening barriers did Pat use during the interaction?
3. If there is anything Pat said that should be different, how would you change it?
4. What listening barriers do you typically use when interacting?
5. What role do non-verbal aspects of communication have in listening?

Inquiry

1. What was the effect of the listening style of Pat upon Mrs Stein?
2. What were the aspects of the situation negatively affecting the listening style of Pat?
3. How might Pat overcome those aspects affecting Mrs Stein?
4. How did Pat demonstrate a commitment to all aspects of Person-centred care?
5. How might you change aspects of this interaction to achieve effective listening?

Action

1. How might healthcare professionals develop their listening skills in practice?
2. List ways of preparing to listen to ensure effective listening.
3. Explain how you would ensure consistently listening in practice.
4. How might you overcome listening barriers to achieve effective listening?
5. Explain how effective listening achieves mutual understanding.

Additional activities

1. Consider situations that might encourage the use of listening barriers.

2. Suggest reasons why these situations might encourage using listening barriers.

3. Suggest ways to overcome the tendency to not listen in such situations.

4. Refer to Chapter 11 of O'Toole, *Communication: Core interpersonal skills for healthcare professionals*, 5th ed. Choose a scenario from Section 4 and allocate the role of healthcare professional and Person. Perform the role play.

5. Reflect on the effectiveness of communication during the role plays to improve performance when interacting in similar circumstances.

   a. Observe and evaluate both effective and ineffective listening.

   b. Observe and evaluate demonstration of all aspects of Step 1 of Person/Family-centred Care: Mutual Understanding: Respect, Empathy and Developing Trust.

   c. Observe and evaluate the verbal messages of the healthcare professional demonstrating aspects of listening.

   d. Observe and evaluate the non-verbal messages of the healthcare professional reflecting aspects of listening.

   e. Observe and evaluate the effectiveness of the listening.

   f. Consider how your thoughts about listening have changed and how to apply this.

   g. Suggest how to improve your listening in all future interactions.

Text link

Chapter 11, 'Awareness of listening to facilitate Person/s-centred communication in healthcare'. In O'Toole, G. (2024). *Communication: Core interpersonal skills for healthcare professionals* (5th ed.). Elsevier.

A FINAL WORD

Effective listening is an important component of Person/Family-centred care. It benefits the Person, the healthcare professional and their employing service. It also contributes to the quality of care and thus the ultimate outcomes for the Person/s. It demonstrates a focus on the Person and their needs. This focus contributes to the satisfaction of the Person and their commitment to following healthcare professional suggestions relating to their needs and, thus, possible improvement. It requires understanding of the personal listening habits of the healthcare professional and awareness of their typical barriers affecting listening. The Person is the focus and not the needs of, or expectations affecting, the healthcare professional. This is essential for satisfying and quality healthcare.

CHAPTER 8

Considering and managing different environments

INTRODUCTION

Healthcare professionals, unless new to a particular service, often assume knowledge of the physical environment of the service. Person/s (and other healthcare professionals) who are new to a physical environment will often experience confusion and an element of uncertainty, until becoming familiar with that environment. There are many aspects contributing to a physical environment including the layout of the overall building (for example, the location of the toilets and treatment rooms) along with the temperature, the lighting, the cleanliness of the environment, the friendliness of the staff, the noise levels and the possibility of distractions. The appearance of the healthcare professional is also a component of the physical environment contributing to the overall effect of the physical environment. There are other relevant environments contributing to effective communication. These include the emotional status of the healthcare professional and the Person; the cultural reality of the healthcare professional and the Person; the sexual environment; the social environments of the healthcare professional and the Person and, finally, the spiritual environments typical to each individual, thereby influencing the interactions within the healthcare process. All these environments require consideration to achieve Person/Family-centred Care and effective communication for all Person/s.

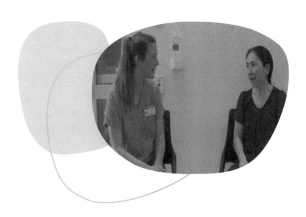

Kim and Charlie's story

 View Kim and Charlie's story or read the transcript.

The Persons: Kim (mother) and Charlie (daughter)

In this story, Kim, the mother of Charlie, does not usually accompany her daughter to receive treatment.

Charlie has a sensory integration disorder relating to processing and managing negative emotions. This results in challenging behaviour (kicking and hitting), often due to unexpected change to usual habits producing negative emotions, including frustration. However, today, unexpected events for the husband and the ability to leave work after lunch made it possible for Kim to bring Charlie for her regular weekly session. Kim does not know anyone from the health service. They have also had to travel by public transport today and this has made them a little late. Not knowing anyone and arriving late creates feelings of stress for Kim. Upon entering the waiting area, Charlie runs to someone, hugging them. Kim assumes this healthcare professional is Pat, who usually sees Charlie for interventions. There is another healthcare professional with Pat called Meg.

After Pat and Charlie go to their usual room, Kim sits for a moment to help her relax. After a short time, Kim and Meg go to a different room to discuss progress and possible improvement. The discussion between Meg and Kim identifies cultural differences and spiritual values specific to this family, including replacing shoes with slippers when entering a house or room and giving thanks for food before eating. These habits are not followed at preschool typically, producing challenging behaviour from Charlie. These expectations have been explained to the staff at the preschool. However, there is inconsistent accommodation of these habits for Charlie, thereby producing frustration for Charlie. Whether or not Charlie has any friends at preschool is unclear. Her upcoming birthday is providing the opportunity to identify possible friends, as invitations to the party will be given to all the children in her class.

Kim indicates, since the implementation of a home program (suggested by Pat), Charlie is more able to control her emotions. This can vary depending on the expectations of her grandparents who live with the family. Charlie loves having them live in their house, despite the challenges for her.

Before ending the conversation, Kim indicates the benefits of discussing Charlie and her needs with someone other than her partner.

The healthcare professional: Meg Smith

There are initially two healthcare professionals. Pat is the healthcare professional regularly treating Charlie. The other, Meg, has an appointment to discuss progress and possible improvement in Charlie. The parent with Charlie today is not the usual one. This creates questions from Pat. However,

Pat notices the stress Kim is experiencing, therefore suggesting she sit for a moment to relax a little. Kim rests and then follows Meg to a room. Upon entering the room, they sit facing each other. Meg asks about the comfort of the chair for Kim. When Kim mentions the heat in the room, Meg responds by opening the window.

They then discuss the improvements in Charlie both at home and at preschool. The discussion indicates improvement at home due to the home program given by Pat. However, things at preschool vary. The preschool is not able to accommodate the removal of the shoes (except when using the trampoline, which Charlie loves), while inconsistently accommodating giving thanks for food before eating. Meg acknowledges that different habits can be difficult for young children, understandably causing frustration for Charlie.

Meg explores the possibility of Charlie having friends at preschool. This exploration leads to discussion of the birthday party for Charlie, and invitations to all the children in her class at preschool. This has the potential to identify if Charlie has any friends at preschool. Meg also asks about managing Charlie during the party in case of biting and hitting. Meg then notes a discussion with both parents has created a plan to manage such behaviour during the party. Meg also says she hopes the party goes well for everyone.

Meg then asks how her parents who live with them manage Charlie and her aggressive outbursts. This leads to indication that Charlie loves living with her grandparents; however, she is not always able to control her emotions or behaviour when they disapprove of her behaviour.

The setting

Location: Initially in the waiting area of an outpatient health service, with two healthcare professionals waiting there. The Persons (Kim and Charlie) meet the two healthcare professionals (Pat and Meg) in the waiting room. After a brief conversation, one healthcare professional, Pat, takes the child, Charlie, into an activity room and the other healthcare professional takes the parent, Kim, into a quiet private room sitting facing each other.

The context: An outpatient service visited by a parent (Kim who is Asian) and a child (Charlie who is mixed race). Charlie and her other parent (Sam) have been attending this service for ongoing treatment (one-hour sessions for eight weeks), seeing the same healthcare professional,

Pat. This week a different healthcare professional, Meg, is seeing them to explore the progress and perceived improvement in the child. Kim is attending for the first time as Sam is sleeping before working an unexpected night shift, so Kim has taken a few hours off work in order to accompany Charlie today.

Physical setting: After the waiting room, the healthcare professional, Meg, and the parent, Kim, are sitting opposite each other in a quiet private space, with Meg holding something on her lap for notetaking.

Reflection

1. What did the healthcare professional, Meg, do to demonstrate respect?
2. Was there any thought about the spiritual environment of the preschool?
3. How would *you* manage the spiritual environments during interactions?
4. What in the interaction related to cultural environments and how were they considered or managed?
5. How would *you* manage variations in cultural environments in practice?

Inquiry

1. How effective was the consideration of the physical environment?
2. How did Meg include consideration of the physical environment in the interaction?
3. How did the healthcare professionals, Meg and Pat, manage the emotional environment at the beginning?
4. How did Meg consider the social environments affecting Kim and Charlie?
5. How did Meg demonstrate a commitment to Person/Family-centred Care?

Action

Remember the healthcare professional does not always have the ability to accommodate all environments in practice, but is able to refer the Person to someone who could accommodate the environment affecting them the most.

1. List the components of environments affecting Person/s in healthcare.
2. Suggest how to accommodate them in practice.
3. List the possible environments affecting healthcare professionals.
4. Suggest how to accommodate them in practice.
5. Consider how you might ensure effective consideration and management of different environments in all interactions whether with Person/s or colleagues.

Additional activities

Refer to Chapter 12 of O'Toole, *Communication: Core interpersonal skills for healthcare professionals*, 5th ed., to complete the following using small group discussion and feedback with the entire class.

1. What might be the typical response from the Person/s if the healthcare professional does not consider the effect of the physical environment on the Person/s when interacting with them?
2. What effect can the current emotional environment (for both or either the Person/s or the healthcare professional) have on the outcome of any interaction?
3. How can the social environments of the Person/s affect their commitment to treatment and thus their improvement?
4. What variations in different cultural environments (both of individual services and those of the Person/s) might affect the healthcare professional in everyday practice?
5. Spiritual environments can vary from culture to culture and within countries, however they will affect expectations. How might the healthcare professional accommodate spiritual environments?

Text link

Chapter 12, 'Awareness of the effects of different environments upon healthcare communication'. In O'Toole, G. (2024). *Communication: Core interpersonal skills for healthcare professionals* (5th ed.). Elsevier.

A FINAL WORD

Consideration and management of all relevant environments when providing healthcare is important. It ensures achievement of Person/Family-centred Care. Some relevant environments might be easy to consider while others are a little more challenging. Certainly, it is easy to consider and manage the physical environments, although sometimes these are unintentionally forgotten. However, consideration of the social and related cultural environments can be more difficult, depending on the awareness and experience of the healthcare professional with these environments. Such environments can affect responses to expectations of the healthcare professional and of the Person/s relating to intervention protocols. Exploration and consideration of these particular environments can produce positive and satisfying outcomes. Similarly, consideration of the emotional environment affecting the Person/s and management of the effect of this environment by the healthcare professional is essential. Such consideration and management can ultimately result in the development of rapport and, thus, a therapeutic relationship. The spiritual environment may have the most profound effect on the Person/s and the healthcare professional. This environment may guide every action and particular daily habits in the life of both the Person/s and the healthcare professional. It is often the most difficult to explore, but typically the most important. It may affect the involvement of the Person/s in their intervention protocols, therefore indicating the need for consideration and, where appropriate, management of this environment. Consideration and management of those environments affecting the Person/s contribute to the quality of care and, thus, satisfying outcomes.

CHAPTER 9
Holistic communication

INTRODUCTION

Communication is often informed by the physical appearance and physical needs of the Person/s. This physical aspect of the Person/s is typically obvious. However, it does not always indicate the realities of other aspects affecting the overall needs of the Person/s. Holistic communication and resultant care requires consideration and often accommodation of all aspects of the Person/s. These aspects include the emotional state and needs of the Person/s (not always obvious); the cognitive abilities and needs, the social and cultural realities with associated needs, the sexual aspect, along with the spiritual aspect of the Person/s and the resultant behaviour. These aspects influence the needs of the Person/s and thus should influence their care. Despite some of these aspects being the direct focus of particular health professions, it is important to consider all aspects of the Person/s when providing healthcare. Such consideration demonstrates respect and empathy, important components of the first step of Person/Family-centred care (P/F-cC), mutual understanding. It also allows the healthcare professional to refer the Person/s to other relevant professionals or facilities. All these aspects affect the wellbeing and ultimate outcomes of any healthcare. Therefore, consideration of all these aspects contributes to the provision of appropriate and satisfactory care from the perspective of the Person/s, thereby contributing to the satisfaction of the healthcare professional and their employer.

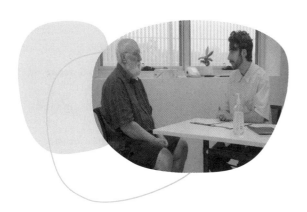

Vic's story

 View Vic's story or read the transcript.

The Person: Vic

In this story, Vic is sitting with a handkerchief wiping his tears. He is crying and obviously upset. A different healthcare professional to the one Vic usually sees enters the room and, despite his distress, when Vic learns about their absence, he expresses concern for them. He is upset because his wife and adult child were recently killed in a car accident. However, this is unknown to the usual healthcare professional as they typically tell Vic that treatment and improvement is more important than anything else, so he should forget what is upsetting him and stop crying.

The current healthcare professional, Glen, indicates he would like to know the cause of the tears. Vic does not believe this healthcare professional is really interested as the usual one has shown no interest. After several questions relating to his upset, Vic eventually trusts this healthcare professional enough to tell him about the loss of his important family members. Vic also says he thought coming for healthcare would make him feel better. It takes him away from his empty house, in which he now feels lonely. The empathic response of Glen encourages Vic to continue talking about his loss and his hope of seeing his wife and child when he dies. When Glen says he will organise a meeting with the Chaplain, Vic expresses gratitude and thanks. He is thankful as Glen has shown interest in his feelings, while also exploring ways to assist him.

The healthcare professional: Glen Collins

Glen is seeing Vic for the first time. He enters the room, introduces himself, confirms the name that Vic prefers and explains the absence of the usual healthcare professional. After checking the medical records about the weekly procedures for Vic, he says he knows what to do with Vic today. He notices how upset Vic appears, asking if Vic is OK. Despite Vic saying he will be OK in a moment, the healthcare professional continues to ask Vic about his emotions. Glen repeatedly demonstrates empathy and concern for Vic. He explores the emotions, consistently expressing his interest and concern.

He asks about the cause of this distress, continuing to encourage Vic to disclose the reasons. Vic is reticent to disclose the cause because of the response of the usual healthcare professional, assuming Glen will have the same reaction. Glen demonstrates he is worthy of trust and Vic eventually explains the cause. Upon hearing about the loss of these important family members he expresses regret about the reaction of the usual healthcare professional, expressing empathy about the loss and understanding about the desire to leave the empty and lonely house to come for treatment. This encourages Vic to indicate the only comfort he has is that he will see them when he

dies. Glen acknowledges the spiritual aspect of Vic, suggesting a meeting with the service Chaplain to assist Vic.

The setting

Location: A quiet private space with chairs and a table. The healthcare professional (Glen) and Vic are facing each other, sitting a comfortable distance apart.

Context: An outpatient service that Vic has been attending for ongoing treatment (1 hour sessions) for a couple of weeks, seeing the same healthcare professional. However, today the regular healthcare professional is away, and a different healthcare professional, Glen, is attending to Vic.

Physical setting: The healthcare professional (Glen) and the Person (Vic) are sitting opposite each other with various types of healthcare equipment in the room.

Reflection

1. What was the effect of the first healthcare professional on Vic?

2. Compare the different effects of the two healthcare professionals on Vic.

3. How did the non-verbal messages of the second healthcare professional, Glen, affect the interaction?

4. Would deeper consideration of particular aspects of the Person be useful? If so, why?

5. How might **you** accommodate the spiritual aspect of the Person in practice?

Inquiry

1. What did the healthcare professional in the video do to develop trust and rapport?

2. What three aspects of the whole Person/s did the healthcare professional consider?

3. How effective was the consideration of the different aspects of the whole Person/s?

4. Was the consideration of the three aspects and the response appropriate? If so, why? If not, why not?

5. How might you change aspects of this interaction to achieve more holistic communication?

Action

1. List the seven aspects of the whole Person/s.
2. Explain how you would consistently consider each aspect of the whole Person/s in practice.
3. Explain why it is important to consider more than the physical aspect of Person/s.
4. Discuss how you accommodate differences to you in the sexual aspect of Person/s.
5. Decide how you can accommodate the differences in the spiritual aspect of Person/s.

Additional activities

1. Refer to Chapters 9 and 13 of O'Toole, *Communication: Core interpersonal skills for healthcare professionals*, 5th ed. Choose a scenario from Section 4 and allocate the role of healthcare professional (HcP) and Person. Perform the role play.
2. Choose a particular aspect of the whole Person and role play how to accommodate that aspect in practice. The 'Person' must decide their personal preferences relating to the chosen aspect. Role plays can be repeated focusing on different aspects of the whole Person.
3. Reflect on the effectiveness of communication during the role plays to improve performance when interacting in similar circumstances.

a. Observe and evaluate both the effective and the ineffective consideration of the chosen aspect during the interaction.
b. Observe and evaluate demonstration of all aspects of Step 1 of Person/Family-centred Care: Mutual Understanding: Respect, Empathy and Developing Trust.
c. Observe and evaluate the verbal messages of the healthcare professional.
d. Observe and evaluate the non-verbal messages of the healthcare professional.
e. Observe and evaluate the effectiveness of the listening.
f. Consider how your thoughts about the different aspects of the whole Person have changed and how to apply this.
g. Suggest how to improve consideration of all aspects of the Person in practice, including referral to the appropriate service or healthcare professional.

Text links

Chapter 9, 'Awareness of the whole "Person/s" for healthcare communication' and Chapter 13, 'Holistic communication contributing to holistic healthcare'. In O'Toole, G. (2024). Communication: Core interpersonal skills for healthcare professionals (5th ed.). Elsevier.

A FINAL WORD

Holistic communication requires consideration of the whole Person/s, not merely a focus on the physical aspect. Particular health professions may focus on a particular aspect of the Person/s, therefore allowing the healthcare professional to feel justified when avoiding consideration of any other aspect. However, ignoring the various aspects of the whole Person/s can result in limitations in the health outcomes. In order to ensure positive and appropriate outcomes, it is essential to consider and accommodate the whole Person/s. Referral to an appropriate service or healthcare professional can facilitate this accommodation. Consideration and accommodation of the whole Person/s results in the overall wellbeing of the Person/s, thereby indicating the importance of considering the whole Person/s. Consideration of the whole Person contributes to both effective communication and Person/Family-centred Care.

CHAPTER 10
Managing misunderstandings and conflict

INTRODUCTION

There is often a relationship between misunderstandings and conflict. A misunderstanding may cause inappropriate or unexpected reactions, thereby producing conflict. Alternatively, conflict and expression of strong negative emotions may cause misunderstandings resulting from the inappropriate communication of the strong negative emotions. There are various methods of managing both conflict and misunderstandings in order to achieve mutual understanding and thus effective communication and quality Person/Family-centred Care. In fact, the presence of conflict and misunderstandings may reduce the level of trust in all interacting individuals. This will therefore affect the possibility of therapeutic relationships and effective collaboration to provide satisfactory and appropriate care. It is important then to ensure appropriate responses to strong negative emotions in order to avoid interactions escalating into aggressive conflict and possible misunderstandings and resultant conflict. Equally important is the need to invest time to ensure the achievement of mutual understanding for all interacting individuals. Important elements for avoiding both of these aspects of communication are reflection about the details of the interaction, exploring how to avoid both conflict and misunderstandings in the future, along with effective listening.

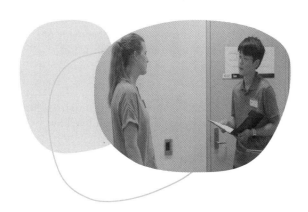

Michael and Meg's story

 View Michael and Meg's story or read the transcript.

Healthcare professional 1: Michael Wang

In this story, one healthcare professional, Michael, leaves a storeroom. He appears unhappy and perhaps a little frustrated. He has just spent five minutes searching for a particular piece of equipment necessary for his next treatment session with a child on the spectrum, with particular sensory-processing needs. This child has particular sensory issues requiring specific colours and types of equipment to ensure effective communication and care.

Upon leaving the storeroom, Michael is met by another healthcare professional, Meg. He expresses his difficulty with limited frustration, but with concern for the child in his next session. He indicates he booked the green and yellow snake earlier that day, as soon as the service opened. Meg suggests several possible alternatives, including the use of a different coloured snake, since they weigh the same.

A discussion follows relating to the needs of the child, the booking of equipment, a team working in remote locations with particular equipment, the fact that Meg is relatively new to the service and the differences in weights of toys. Michael tells Meg that she needs to take responsibility for learning about particular details relating to the staff and service procedures.

Notice: while feeling frustrated, Michael appropriately controls his emotions to assist in avoiding unnecessary conflict.

Healthcare professional 2: Meg Smith

Healthcare professional Meg appears very sure that she is right, despite appearing a little insecure and frustrated. She indicates a lack of understanding about the need for a specific colour of weighted snake. She suggests Michael use the other coloured snake, indicating limited care or understanding about the need of his client. She mentions remembering a comment by a colleague relating to the green and yellow snake. She is however unsure about when they had that conversation or in fact who the colleague was that indicated they would be taking it offsite. Her non-verbal messages throughout the interaction suggest frustration and not understanding the problem.

The setting

This video relates to a paediatric service, providing interventions for children and adolescents with sensory-processing disorders. One of the useful interventions for such children is the use of weighted toys. These weighted toys are often snakes, dogs, turtles and other animals typically known by children. The weight of these toys varies (approximately 500 g to 2.2 kg) depending on the sensory needs of the child.

Location: Just outside a storeroom in a multiprofessional paediatric community health service, where the necessary healthcare equipment is stored and labelled on shelves or in appropriate spaces. This storeroom stores different kinds of paediatric equipment.

Context: Healthcare services typically store the required equipment in rooms with shelves and/or spaces for placing the equipment. The shelves and spaces are usually labelled, to indicate where to find and/or return specific items. It is also common for such storerooms to require the individual taking the equipment to sign and date the time they take it and the time and date they return it.

On the storeroom door is a sign saying:

REMEMBER to sign & date when taking equipment and when returning it.

Please return ALL Equipment to its original place. THANKS

Physical setting: Outside the storeroom of a paediatric health service.

Reflection

1. How do you manage misunderstandings when you have misunderstood someone?

2. How can you improve your management of your misunderstanding to achieve effective communication?

3. How do you manage misunderstandings when someone else has misunderstood you?

4. How do you manage differences in opinion about things you are sure you understand?

5. How can you improve your management of differences in opinion during healthcare?

Inquiry

1. How did Michael manage the misunderstanding about the location of the green and yellow snake?

2. Explain why this was an effective method of managing a misunderstanding.

3. How did both the healthcare professionals demonstrate respect for each other?

4. What made management of the disagreement effective, thereby avoiding conflict?

5. How might you change aspects of this interaction to achieve more effective communication when experiencing misunderstandings?

Action

1. List the possible reasons for misunderstandings.

2. Explain how you would consistently avoid misunderstandings in practice.

3. Consider and explain the role and relevance of emotional control when experiencing clashes during interactions.

4. Decide how you can consistently avoid conflict during interactions in practice.

5. Consider how you might ensure mutual understanding when experiencing conflict.

Additional activities

1. Refer to Chapters 14, 15 and 18 of O'Toole, Communication: Core interpersonal skills for healthcare professionals, 5th ed. Choose a scenario from Section 4 and allocate the role of healthcare professional (HcP) and Person. Perform the role play.

2. Reflect on the effectiveness of communication during the role plays to improve performance when experiencing misunderstandings.

   a. Observe and evaluate both the effective and the ineffective aspects of the misunderstanding.

   b. Observe and evaluate demonstration of all aspects of Step 1 of Person/Family-centred Care: Mutual Understanding: Respect, Empathy and Developing Trust.

   c. Observe and evaluate the verbal messages of each individual during the role play.

   d. Observe and evaluate the non-verbal messages of the individual playing the healthcare professional.

   e. Observe and evaluate the effectiveness of the listening of each individual.

   f. Consider how your thoughts about misunderstandings have changed and how to apply this difference in practice.

   g. Suggest how to improve all future interactions with misunderstandings.

3. Choose a different scenario from Section 4, assign roles, with each individual deciding how to experience conflict during the role play, without discussing their ideas with the other people in the role play.

4. Reflect on the effectiveness of communication during the role plays to improve performance when experiencing conflict.

   a. Observe and evaluate both the effective and the ineffective aspects of communication during the conflict.

   b. Observe and evaluate demonstration or lack of all aspects of Step 1 of Person/Family-centred Care: Mutual Understanding: Respect, Empathy and Developing Trust during the interaction.

   c. Observe and evaluate the verbal messages of each individual during the role play.

   d. Observe and evaluate the non-verbal messages of the individual playing the healthcare professional.

   e. Observe and evaluate the effectiveness of the listening of each individual.

   f. Consider how your thoughts about misunderstandings have changed and how to apply this difference in practice.

   g. Suggest how to improve all future interactions with misunderstandings.

Text links

Chapter 14, 'Effective interpersonal communication within multidisciplinary teams', Chapter 15, 'Managing conflict when communicating as a healthcare professional' and Chapter 18, 'Misunderstandings and communication for the healthcare professional'. In O'Toole, G. (2024). *Communication: Core interpersonal skills for healthcare professionals* (5th ed.). Elsevier.

A FINAL WORD

The realities of life may result in misunderstandings and conflict (although there is not always a connection). The occurrence of misunderstandings and conflict in healthcare, however, can result in the reduction of trust in all relationships occurring in this setting, along with a reduction in the satisfaction levels and quality of care. Wherever possible it is essential that the healthcare professional strives to avoid misunderstandings and possible conflict. The role of emotions in such situations is important. Emotions can either increase or avoid both misunderstandings and conflict. Reflection is a necessary means of increasing self-awareness and thus avoiding both. Such reflection will assist the healthcare professional to identify the causes of misunderstandings and also their typical responses in conflict situations. Some responses may intensify the conflict and others can decrease and expel any conflict. Awareness of the causes and circumstances producing misunderstandings and conflict is therefore an essential skill for all healthcare professionals.

CHAPTER 11

Telehealth or telecommunication to deliver healthcare

INTRODUCTION

Telehealth or telecommunication uses an online video connection to connect the Person/s and the healthcare professional. This video connection is possible through devices with cameras and reliable internet connections. It has typically been used with Person/s living in rural and remote areas or with Person/s experiencing chronic disorders or reduced mobility. It has more recently become a regular way of providing health care because of the Coronavirus (COVID-19) pandemic. A video consultation has the potential to provide safe and equitable care for all. It also reduces the possibility of infection when managing infectious diseases. This kind of care does, however, require financial investment in relevant devices and services; security of data transmission; secure and reliable internet access and also secure data storage, with secure back-up and disposal methods. Knowledge of these levels of security encourage relevant Person/s to engage and connect using a video internet connection. However, it requires appropriate security measures and trained healthcare professionals to effectively use the technology and to problem solve (trouble shoot) when necessary. In some circumstances it may require training of the Person/s using this interface, to ensure their ability to connect and effectively use their devices. Services offering telehealth typically employ able technical experts to manage and maintain the devices and the interface necessary for this mode of healthcare delivery. Telehealth is a consistent method of providing safe and satisfying care in particular circumstances.

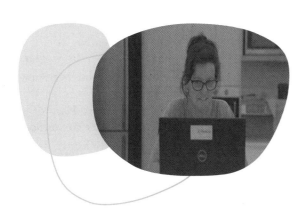

Julien's story

 View Julien's story or read the transcript.

The Person: Julien

In this story, Julien obviously enjoys and appreciates the regular connection with the healthcare professional,

Meg, and her suggestions, equipment provision and encouragement, along with her consideration when experiencing difficulty connecting remotely.

Julien demonstrated increased movement in both her arm and leg, indicating her commitment to appropriate regular exercise, use of provided equipment along with a need to decrease her level of pain. Julien does, however, express reticence about one particular exercise. She acknowledges that this particular exercise will improve her function. However, she expresses fear of increased levels of pain in her knee if doing this exercise.

Overall Julien appears satisfied with her care, despite it being online and the sometimes unreliable nature of internet connections.

The healthcare professional: Meg Smith

Meg, the healthcare professional, greets the Person, Julien, with apologies and explanation about connection difficulties (not unusual with internet usage for communication). Her interaction with Julien demonstrates all aspects of Person/Family-centred Care and awareness of the importance of all aspects of communication when using online, electronic visual and auditory methods (telehealth/telecommunication).

Meg explores the elements of Julien's improvement, including consideration of regularly completing the relevant exercises; her pain levels; movement of her arm and knee, appropriate methods of dressing, toileting, showering, bed height and use of the associated equipment.

Meg answers a question relating to a needed piece of equipment with an indication of continued focus on the details of the question to facilitate a quick response for Julien. She also discusses sleeping, something difficult for Julien due to pain. Meg stresses the importance of sleep for recovery.

Before ending the session, Meg mentions future online appointments and the need to continue regularly doing the prescribed exercises.

The setting

Location: Quiet private room with a table. There is a computer with a camera on the table, with a comfortable chair for the healthcare professional, Meg. There is appropriate lighting and noise regulation. The Person, Julien, is sitting in her kitchen. The camera may be inbuilt or external.

Context: A healthcare service offering care for individuals unable to attend the service. Trained healthcare professionals are able to connect with the Person/s using video and secure/encrypted internet access.

Physical setting: The healthcare professional, Meg, has a secure, online connection with the Person, Julien. They are connecting using devices designed to provide video and audio connection. They both see the other on their screens.

Reflection

1. What did the healthcare professional, Meg, do to demonstrate respect?

2. Is there is anything Meg said that should be different? How would you change it?

3. How did the non-verbal messages of Meg affect the interaction?

4. When using telecommunication, what would **you** need to do to ensure Person/Family-centred-Care?

5. When using telecommunication, what would **you** need to do to achieve effective communication?

Inquiry

1. How effective was the interaction using technical devices to connect?

2. What did Meg do to develop trust and rapport?

3. How did Meg demonstrate a commitment to Person/Family-centred Care?

4. How did Meg demonstrate effective listening throughout the interaction?

5. How might you change aspects of this interaction to increase effective communication?

Action

1. What is required when using telehealth to deliver healthcare?

2. Explain how you would consistently demonstrate respect during a telehealth session.

3. Write a list of required actions before beginning a telehealth session.

4. Decide how to trouble shoot for the Person/s if they are having difficulty with their connection.

5. Consider how you might ensure effective collaboration when using telehealth.

Additional activities

Refer to Chapter 21 of O'Toole, *Communication: Core interpersonal skills for healthcare professionals*, 5th ed. In groups, answer the following questions. When completed, share the answers with the large group.

a. List the requirements of telehealth/telecommunication in healthcare.

b. Discuss the possible difficulties of your health profession if using telehealth.

c. Consider and summarise the relevant guidelines for the use of telehealth in your location.

d. Decide how to consistently conform to these guidelines when using telehealth.

e. Consider and make decisions about the content for the training of a healthcare professional to empower them to effectively use telehealth.

Text link

Chapter 21, 'Remote telecommunication or telehealth: 2 The seen, but not-in-the-room healthcare professional'. In O'Toole, G. (2024). *Communication: Core interpersonal skills for healthcare professionals* (5th ed.). Elsevier.

A FINAL WORD

Telehealth or telecommunication can provide cost-effective and appropriate healthcare for remote Person/s or those with chronic disorders or conditions reducing mobility. It allows a healthcare professional to see the Person/s despite being in different locations, rather than travelling large distances to visit in-person. The cost of the travel can be redirected to purchase the necessary equipment and staff for telehealth connections. This type of connection allows the healthcare professional and the Person/s to not only see each other, but also observe the non-verbal messages and movements of each other, thereby enhancing the quality of the interaction. Training in the use of the required equipment and possible methods of solving problems is beneficial for all, thereby reducing possible anxiety or frustration relating to technical difficulties. It is also important to ensure secure connection to avoid inappropriate interruptions or exploration of personal health records. While learning to use telehealth and ensuring security for all requires care, focus and planning, telehealth has the advantage of interacting in a visual interface, thereby encouraging effective communication.

CHAPTER 12

Using personal social media and the healthcare professional

INTRODUCTION

Social media has a worldwide presence today. Many people use it to connect with friends and family, regardless of their location (sometimes even if sitting in the same room!). Technology and improved devices make the use of social media to connect with others possible in many situations and locations. However, it is a connection that is not in-person. This has many potential consequences. The person sending the messages, being unable to see or experience the responses of those receiving the messages, does not typically adjust their messages to accommodate the responses of the audience. This is acceptable if the responses are positive. However, someone in the audience may be negatively affected by the content of the message. If communicating in-person, the sender of the message is able to identify the effect and respond to, encourage or comfort them or explain the meaning of the message to reduce the negative effects. Communicating through social media does not allow this to occur for the sender or the receivers of the messages. Therefore, achieving effective and appropriate communication through social media requires thought and consideration before sending the written message.

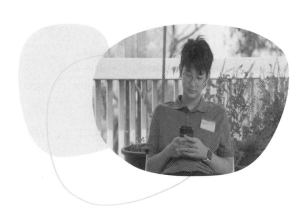

Michael's story

 View Michael's story or read the transcript.

The healthcare professional: Michael Wang (aka Sadi)

In this story, Michael has just arrived home. He relaxes on the deck at home after a busy day at work.

He typically uses social media to express his feelings with the people in his chat.

Today he expresses ongoing frustration with people assuming he is too young to be a qualified healthcare professional. He indicates he is 'sick' of people assuming he should still be at school!

The friends reply by saying it is a compliment, indicating he should NOT be upset. The comments repeat this idea.

Michael then mentions one of his Person/s, including their name. He indicates that he made a comment to this Person about their age in response to their comment about his own age. This Person is a well-known newsreader – all the friends then make comments relating to this Person/s. Michael provides information about this Person and their injury and resulting level of function. These entries lead to the mention of the date of birth (DoB) of the Person. The friends respond with the idea of sending the newsreader birthday wishes on the right date.

The setting

Location: Home of the healthcare professional, Michael, on the outside deck, with his mobile phone.

Context: Michael has just returned from work, is now at home, still in uniform with his name badge still on, looking at his mobile phone.

Physical setting: An outside area with appropriate light and a comfortable chair.

Reflection

1. If you were the Person/s, how would you feel if personal details were entered onto the social media interface of your healthcare professional?

2. How would you, as the Person/s, respond to the healthcare professional?

3. How could Michael respond to the questions asked by his friends on the chat?

4. As many individuals are often befriended or are able to 'hack into' personal social media chats, what are the legal implications of the recorded details in this chat?

5. Consider the implications for Michael resulting from his entries in this chat.

Inquiry

1. How appropriate was the use of the name of the Person in this chat? Why or why not?

2. How do you think the use of the name of the Person might affect the reputation of Michael?

3. How appropriate was the mention of the specific condition of the Person in this chat? Why or why not?

4. How appropriate was disclosing the date of birth of the Person in this chat? Why or why not?

5. How might you change aspects of this interaction to achieve appropriate entries on social media?

Action

1. List the components of the guidelines for use of social media (typically in Codes of Conduct) relevant to your health profession.

2. Explain how you would consistently achieve these on personal social media.

3. Some healthcare services use social media to communicate with the Person/s. If working for such a healthcare service, how would you ensure differentiation between the professional and personal interface of social media?

4. Write a list of things to remember when using personal social media.

5. Consider how you might ensure appropriate use of personal social media if you are working as a healthcare professional.

Additional activities

Refer to Chapters 19 and 23 of O'Toole, *Communication: Core interpersonal skills for healthcare professionals*, 5th ed. Consider the following in a group discussion about entries in personal social media.

a. Consider the ethical requirement of working as a healthcare professional and how they apply to the personal use of social media (relevant Code of Conduct or Workplace Ethics).

b. Consider how and why it is easy to misunderstand when using social media.

c. Decide how to ensure effective communication when using personal social media.

d. What can you do to ensure any future employees exploring your social media entries would be willing to employ you?

e. Consider and explain the increased suicide rates in young people since the existence of social media (see Bannink et al., 2014; Brunstein Klomek et al., 2010).

Text links

Chapter 19, 'Ethical communication in healthcare' and Chapter 23 'Social media or "not present in person" communication and the healthcare professional'. In O'Toole, G. (2024). *Communication: Core interpersonal skills for healthcare professionals* (5th ed.). Elsevier.

A FINAL WORD

Social media is a common phenomenon today. Many people use it as their usual form of connection with others around the world. Evidence, however, suggests this connection is superficial with a greater focus on the sender of the message and their feelings than the feelings or life of anyone else. It seems then to require healthcare professionals to take care when using social media for personal use. Consideration of the content and possible meaning of any messages is essential, whether using social media for professional or for social communication. The intent of the message also requires consideration. If to complain or to malign another individual, it is important to consider the possible effects both personally and professionally for the healthcare professional, but also for those reading the messages. Expression of negative emotions on social media (especially relating to Person/s) may increase the intensity of the feelings for both the sender and the receivers of the message rather than decrease them. It may also affect the achievement of Person/Family-centred Care with that individual, and possibly other Person/s. Careful and thoughtful use of social media is important for any healthcare professional, thereby achieving effective and appropriate communication. This will have a positive effect on the reputation of the healthcare professional and thus the satisfaction relating to the quality of their healthcare.

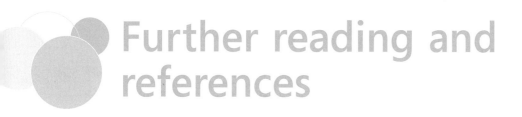

Further reading and references

Chapter 1

FURTHER READING

Davis, C. M., & Musolino, G. M. (2016). *Patient practitioner interaction: An experiential manual for developing the art of healthcare* (6th ed.). SLACK.

Granger, K. (2013). Healthcare staff must properly introduce themselves to patients. *BMJ, 347*(f), 5833. https://doi.org/10.1136/bmj.f5833.

Guest, M. (2016). How to introduce yourself to patients. *Nursing Standard, 30*(41), 36–38. https://doi.org/10.7748/ns.30.41.36.s43.

Honeycutt, A. (2023). *Understanding human behavior: A guide for healthcare professionals* (10th ed.). Cengage Delmar.

McCorry, L. K., & Mason, J. (2019). *Communication skills for the healthcare professionals* (2nd ed.). Jones & Bartlett.

Stein-Parbury, J. (2021). *Patient & person: Interpersonal skills in nursing* (7th ed.). Elsevier.

Chapter 2

FURTHER READING

Beesley, P., Watts, M., & Harrison, M. (2018). *Developing your communication skills in social work*. Sage.

Burrus, A. E., & Willis, L. B. (2022). *Professional communication in speech-language pathology: How to write, talk and act like a clinician* (4th ed.). Plural.

Davis, C. M., & Musolino, G. M. (2016). *Patient practitioner interaction: An experiential manual for developing the art of healthcare* (6th ed.). SLACK.

Devito, J. A. (2021). *The interpersonal communication book* (16th ed.). Pearson.

Egan, G., & Reese, R. J. (2019). *The skilled helper: A problem management and opportunity approach to helping* (11th ed.). Cengage.

Giroldi, E., Veldhuijzen, W., de Leve, T., van der Weijden, T., Bueving, H., & van der Vleuten, C. (2015). 'I still have no idea why this patient was here': An exploration of the difficulties GP trainees experience when gathering information. *Patient Education and Counseling, 98*(7), 837–842.

Haddad, A. M., Purtilo, R. B., & Doherty, R. F. (2019). *Health professional and patient interaction* (9th ed.). Elsevier/Saunders.

Holli, B. B., & Beto, J. A. (2022). *Nutrition counselling and education skills for dietetics professionals* (8th ed.). Lippincott, Williams & Wilkins.

Honeycutt, A., & Milliken, M. A. (2018). *Understanding human behavior: A guide for healthcare providers* (9th ed.). Cengage Delmar.

Stein-Parbury, J. (2021). *Patient and person: Interpersonal skills in nursing* (7th ed.). Elsevier.

Chapter 3

FURTHER READING

Beesley, P., Watts, M., & Harrison, M. (2018). *Developing your communication skills in social work*. Sage.

Egan, G., & Reese, R. J. (2019). *The skilled helper: A problem management and opportunity approach to helping* (11th ed.). Cengage.

Healy, K. (2018). *The skilled communicator in social work: The art and science of communication in practice*. Palgrave.

Henderson, A. (2019). *Communication for health care practice*. Oxford University Press.

Moss, B. (2020). *Communication skills in health and social care* (5th ed.). Sage.

Stein-Parbury, J. (2021). *Patient & person: Interpersonal skills in nursing* (7th ed.). Elsevier.

Chapter 4

REFERENCES

Boud, D., Keogh, R., & Walker, D. (1985). *Reflection: Turning experience into learning*. Kogan Page.

Fish, D., Twinn, S., & Purr, B. (1991). *Improving the supervision of practice in health: Training notes*. West London Institute of Higher Education.

Gibbs, G. (1988). *Learning by doing: A guide to teaching and learning methods. Further Education Unit*. Oxford Polytechnic.

Johns, C. (Ed.). (2022). *Becoming a reflective practitioner* (6th ed.). John Wiley & Sons.

Kolb, D. A. (1984). *Experiential learning*. Prentice Hall.

O'Toole, G. (2024). *Communication: Core interpersonal skills for health professionals* (5th ed.). Churchill Livingstone Elsevier.

Chapter 5

FURTHER READING

Abdou, C. M., & Fingerhut, A. W. (2014). Stereotype threat among black and white women in health care settings. *Cultural Diversity and Ethnic Minority Psychology, 20*(3), 316–323.

Abdou, C. M., Fingerhut, A. W., Jackson, J. S., & Wheaton, F. (2016). Healthcare stereotype threat in older adults in the health and retirement study. *American Journal of Preventive Medicine, 50*(2), 191–198.

Egan, G., & Reese, R. J. (2019). *The skilled helper: A problem management and opportunity approach to helping* (11th ed.). Cengage.

Haddad, A. M., Purtilo, R. B., & Doherty, R. F. (2019). *Health professional and patient interaction* (9th ed.). Elsevier/Saunders.

Honeycutt, A., & Milliken, M. A. (2018). *Understanding human behavior: A guide for healthcare professionals* (9th ed.). Cengage.

Johnson, R., & Withers, M. (2018). Cultural competence in the emergency department: Clinicians as cultural learners. *Emergency Medicine Australasia, 30*, 854–856.

Knapp, M., Hall, J., & Horgan, T. G. (2021). *Nonverbal communication in human interaction* (9th ed.). Kendall Hunt.

Moss, B. (2020). *Communication skills in health and social care* (5th ed.). Sage.

Passi, N. (2018). Looking forward, looking back: An indigenous trainee perspective. *Emergency Medicine Australasia, 30*, 862–863.

Stein-Parbury, J. (2021). *Patient & person: Interpersonal skills in nursing* (7th ed.). Elsevier.

Chapter 6

FURTHER READING

Beesley, P., Watts, M., & Harrison, M. (2018). *Developing your communication skills in social work*. Sage.

Devito, J. A. (2021). *The interpersonal communication book* (16th ed.). Pearson.

Egan, G., & Reese, R. J. (2019). *The skilled helper: A problem management and opportunity approach to helping* (11th ed.). Cengage.

Haddad, A. M., Purtilo, R. B., & Doherty, R. F. (2019). *Health professional and patient interaction* (9th ed.). Elsevier/Saunders.

Harms, L. (2015). *Working with people: Communication skills for reflective practice* (2nd ed.). Oxford University Press.

Henderson, A. (2019). *Communication for health care practice*. Oxford University Press.

Knapp, M., Hall, J., & Horgan, T. G. (2021). *Nonverbal communication in human interaction* (9th ed.). Kendall Hunt.

Stein-Parbury, J. (2021). *Patient & person: Interpersonal skills in nursing* (7th ed.). Elsevier.

Chapter 7

FURTHER READING

Beesley, P., Watts, M., & Harrison, M. (2018). *Developing your communication skills in social work*. Sage.

Bodie, G. D., Keaton, S. A., & Jones, S. M. (2018). Individual listening values moderate the impact of verbal person centeredness on helper evaluations: A test of the dual-process theory of supportive message outcomes. *International Journal of Listening, 32*(3), 217–319. https://doi.org/10.1080/10904018.2016.1194207.

Burrus, A. E., & Willis, L. B. (2022). *Professional communication in speech-language pathology: How to write, talk and act like a clinician* (4th ed.). Plural.

Davis, C. M., & Musolino, G. M. (2016). *Patient practitioner interaction: An experiential manual for developing the art of healthcare* (6th ed.). SLACK.

Honeycutt, A., & Milliken, M. A. (2018). *Understanding human behavior: A guide for healthcare professionals* (9th ed.). Cengage.

Mendes, A. (2020). Communication in care: The importance of soft skills. *Nursing and Residential Care, 22*(9). https://doi.org/10.12968/nrec.2020.22.9.4.

Myers, K. K., Krepper, R., Nibert, A., & Toms, R. (2020). Nurses' active empathic listening behaviours from the voice of the patient. *Nursing Economics, 38*(5), 267–275.

Stein-Parbury, J. (2021). *Patient & person: Interpersonal skills in nursing* (7th ed.). Elsevier.

Chapter 8

FURTHER READING

Egan, G., & Reese, R. J. (2019). *The skilled helper: A problem management and opportunity approach to helping* (11th ed.). Cengage.

Haddad, A. M., Purtilo, R. B., & Doherty, R. F. (2019). *Health professional and patient interaction* (9th ed.). Elsevier/Saunders.

Henderson, A. (2019). *Communication for health care practice*. Oxford University Press.

Honeycutt, A., & Milliken, M. A. (2018). *Understanding human behavior: A guide for healthcare professionals* (9th ed.). Cengage.

Moss, B. (2020). *Communication skills in health and social care* (5th ed.). Sage.

O'Toole, G., & Ramugondo, E. (2018). Occupational therapy and spiritual care. In Carey, L. B., & Mathisen, B. (Eds.), *Spiritual care in allied health practice*. Jessica Kingsley.

Chapter 9

FURTHER READING

Davis, C. M., & Musolino, G. M. (2016). *Patient practitioner interaction: An experiential manual for developing the art of healthcare* (6th ed.). SLACK.

Egan, G., & Reese, R. J. (2019). *The skilled helper: A problem management and opportunity approach to helping* (11th ed.). Cengage.

Falkenheimer, S. A. (2018). Prime: Partnerships in international medical educational: An oral history of the development of an international network in whole person medicine and whole person teaching. *Ethics and Medicine, 34*(2), 87–102.

Haddad, A. M., Purtilo, R. B., & Doherty, R. F. (2019). *Health professional and patient interaction* (9th ed.). Elsevier/Saunders.

Moss, B. (2020). *Communication skills in health and social care* (5th ed.). Sage.

Rosa, W., Hope, S., & Matzo, M. (2019). A holistic stance on entheogens, healing and spiritual care. *Journal of Holistic Nursing, 37*(1), 100–106.

Stein-Parbury, J. (2021). *Patient & person: Interpersonal skills in nursing* (7th ed.). Elsevier.

Chapter 10

FURTHER READING

Davis, C. M., & Musolino, G. M. (2016). *Patient practitioner interaction: An experiential manual for developing the art of healthcare* (6th ed.). SLACK.

Delaney, L. J. (2018). Patient-centred care as an approach to improve health care in Australia. *Collegian, 25*(1), 119–128.

Devito, J. A. (2021). *The interpersonal communication book* (16th ed.). Pearson.

Henderson, A. (2019). *Communication for health care practice*. Oxford University Press.

Honeycutt, A., & Milliken, M. A. (2018). *Understanding human behavior: A guide for healthcare professionals* (9th ed.). Cengage.

McCorry, L. K., & Mason, J. (2019). *Communication skills for the healthcare professionals* (2nd ed.). Jones & Bartlett.

Moss, B. (2020). *Communication skills in health and social care* (5th ed.). Sage.

Stein-Parbury, J. (2021). *Patient & person: Interpersonal skills in nursing* (7th ed.). Elsevier.

Chapter 11

FURTHER READING

Allied Health Professions Australia (AHPA). (2020). Telehealth guide for allied health professionals. AHPA.

Australian College of Rural and Remote Medicine (ACRRM). (2012). *Connecting health services with the future: Guidance on security and privacy issues for clinicians*. ACRRM.

Campbell, J., Theodoros, D., Russell, T., Gillespie, N., & Hartley, N. (2019). Client, provider and community referrer perceptions of telehealth for the delivery of rural paediatric allied health services. *Australian Journal of Rural Health, 27*(5), 419–426.

Choi, A., & Oakley, A. (2021). A retrospective review of cutaneous vascular lesions referred to a teledermatology clinic. *Journal of Primary Health Care, 13*(1), 70–74.

Dudley, S. (2018). The benefits of using tele-practice to support rural families. *Connections, 15*(2), 12.

Fisk, M., Livingstone, A., & Pit, S. W. (2020). Telehealth in the context of COVID-19: Changing perspectives in Australia, the United Kingdom and the United States. *Journal of Medical Internet Research, 22*(6), e19264.

Henderson, A. (2019). *Communication for health care practice*. Oxford University Press.

Henry, B. V., Ames, L. J., Block, D. E., & Vozenilek, J. A. (2018). Experienced practitioners' views on interpersonal skills in telehealth delivery. *Internet Journal of Allied Health Sciences and Practice, 16*(2), Article 2.

Kamei, T., Kanamori, T., & Porter, S. E. (2018). Detection of early-stage changes in people with chronic diseases: A telehome monitoring-based telenursing feasibility study. *Nursing in Health Science, 20*, 313–322.

Moss, B. (2020). *Communication skills in health and social care* (5th ed.). Sage.

Speyer, R., Denman, D., Wilkes-Gillan, S., Chen, Y.-W., Bogaardt, H., Kim, J.-H., Heckathorn, D.-E., & Cordier, R. (2018). Effects of telehealth by allied health professionals and nurses in rural and remote areas: A systematic review and meta-analysis. *Journal of Rehabilitation Medicine, 50*(3), 225–235.

van Houwelingen, T., Ettema, R. G. A., Bleijenberg, N., van Os-Medendorp, H., Kort, H. S. M., & Cate, O. T. (2021). Educational intervention to increase nurses' knowledge self-efficacy and usage of telehealth: A multi-setting pretest-post-test study. *Nurse Education in Practice, 51*, 102924.

Chapter 12

REFERENCES

Bannink, R., Broeren, S., van de Looij-Jansen, P. M., de Waart, F. G., & Raat, H. (2014). Cyber and traditional bullying victimization as a risk factor for mental health problems and suicidal ideation in adolescents. *PLoS ONE, 9*(4), 1–8.

Brunstein Klomek, A., Sourander, A., & Gould, M. (2010). The association of suicide and bullying in childhood to young adults: A review of cross-sectional and longitudinal research findings. *Canadian Journal of Psychiatry, 55*, 282–288.

FURTHER READING

Australian Health Professional Regulation Agency (Ahpra). (2019). Social media policy. www.ahpra.gov.au/ Publications/Social-media-guidance.aspx

Carpiniello, B., & Wasserman, D. (2020). European Psychiatric Association policy paper on ethical aspects in communication with patients and their families. *European Psychiatry, 63*(1), e36, 1–7.

Fischer-Grönlund, C., Brännström, M., & Zingmark, K. (2021). The 'one to five' method – A tool for ethical communication in groups among healthcare professionals. *Nurse Education in Practice, 51*, 102998.

Henderson, M., & Dahnke, M. D. (2015). The ethical use of social media in nursing practice. *Medical–Surgical Nursing, 24*(1), 62–64.

Hjorth, L., & Hinton, S. (2019). *Understanding social media* (2nd ed.). Sage.

Honeycutt, A., & Milliken, M. A. (2021). *Understanding human behavior: A guide for healthcare professionals* (10th ed). Cengage Learning.

Kuss, D. J., & Griffiths, M. D. (2017). Social networking sites and addiction: Ten lessons learnt. *International Journal of Environmental Research and Public Health, 14*, 311.

Long, N. D. (2018). The good, the bad and the ugly of social media: How to navigate through the noise. *Emergency Medicine Australasia, 30*(3), 412–413.

McCallion, M., & McCallion, K. (2021). Reflections on social media. *Academia Letters, article, 329.* https://doi.org/10.20935/AL329.

Moss, B. (2020). *Communication skills in health and social care* (5th ed.). Sage.

Stein-Parbury, J. (2021). *Patient & person: Interpersonal skills in nursing* (7th ed.). Elsevier.

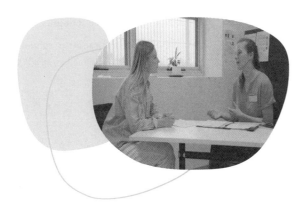

CHAPTER 1

Joan's story

Healthcare Professional (HcP) Meg Smith (Occupational Therapist): Hello, Mrs Thomas, if you'd like to have a seat here?

Mrs Thomas: Thank you.

HcP Meg: Hello, Mrs Thomas. My name is Meg Smith. I would be OK if I called you Mrs Thomas or would you like me to call you something else?

Mrs Thomas: Nice to meet you, Meg. I would prefer Joan.

HcP Meg: OK Joan, I'm an Occupational Therapist and I'll be seeing you to help you manage your daily life with bilateral osteoarthritis – any difficulties you might experience when doing these activities because of pain in your knees?

Joan: Hmmm. I have been a dancer for 10 years and the complications I got from that, but what is an Occupational Therapist and how can you help me?

HcP Meg: That's a good question, Joan. An Occupational Therapist focuses on you as independently and safely as possible doing the activities you need or want to do during your daily life – things like making your meals, going shopping and getting dressed, putting on your shoes and so forth. An Occupational Therapist helps you to do these activities safely and independently. Do you have any questions about this?

Joan: No, not at the moment.

HcP Meg: Well, if you have a question later, please ask me, so we can make sure we understand each other. However, to help you, here are some details regarding our service including my role and there's a toilet just down the hall to the right, if you need it. It's an accessible toilet and it's higher than usual with rails which you might find easier to use. All right. Let me check some details. It says here that you're 34?

Joan: Yep, but I will have my birthday next week, so I will be 35!

HcP Meg: Oh yeah, I see your Date of Birth here. Happy Birthday! Are you doing anything to celebrate?

Joan: Oh, my family is taking me to my favourite restaurant.

HcP Meg: Oh, lovely. And I see that you live with your husband in Riverdale.

Joan: Yep, we've lived there for 10 years now and we don't want to move!

HcP Meg: That's understandable. And I understand you have been having some more pain in your knees.

Joan: Yes, a lot more – so getting up our front stairs has been quite difficult. I'm getting a lot of pain and it takes me quite a long time to get up.

HcP Meg: Oh, you have stairs at home. Did you know you can get a stair lift that will take you up and down the stairs – they're easy to operate and can be folded up to allow other people to use the stairs comfortably and safely.

Joan: I didn't, but how can I get one of those and how much is it?

HcP Meg: I can organise one for you. The cost varies depending on the type, but we can look into that together.

Joan: I also enjoy gardening – is there anything you can do to help me with that?

HcP Meg: Yes, there's a variety of pieces of equipment to help you with the gardening. We can definitely explore those options.

Joan: That would be good. I'm just having trouble getting in and out of bed, it's just too low.

HcP Meg: That's not unusual with pain in knees, there are bed raisers that can raise the bed to a comfortable and safe height to make it easier for you to get in and out of bed. How about the toilet, how do you find getting on and off the toilet?

Joan: Well, the ensuite in my house is quite difficult to use – but I do use the basin to help me up sometimes.

HcP Meg: It's understandable that you use the basin, but that can be quite unsafe. There's toilet seat raisers to raise the height of the toilet to make it easier for you to get on and off the toilet. It can be easily removed for your husband if he doesn't want to use it.

Joan: That sounds great. How quickly can I buy one of those?

HcP Meg: I can see if we have one in stock. If not I can order one for you.

Joan: I'd appreciate that.

HcP Meg: Um, OK one of the things I can do is come to your home to check and ensure your safety and independence at home. Um and it would also be good for you to see a physiotherapist. Have you seen a physiotherapist before to develop your muscle strength with your leg muscles?

Joan: Yeah. I used to see one, but I am not currently.

HcP Meg: OK. Great. I'll refer you to a physio, we have several on staff here – I'll do that as soon as possible. Do you have any questions?

Joan: Perfect, no questions, thank you.

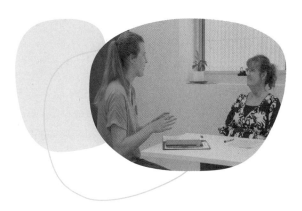

CHAPTER 2

Mrs Richards' story

Healthcare Professional (HcP) Meg Smith: Hello, Mrs Richards. How are you today?

Mrs Richards: Great, thanks. How are you?

HcP Meg: That's good. Doing well. Did you have you any questions after last time we met?

Mrs Richards: Yes, I was just wondering how long I need to be coming to see you for? I know that I will see you for an hour – but I was wondering how many weeks it will be that I'll have to keep seeing you?

HcP Meg: That's a good question – I'm not able to answer it. It will depend on how you respond and your level of improvement.

Mrs Richards: Sure.

HcP Meg: Well, thank you for seeing me today. Before I assess your current abilities and we do some treatment, I have some questions to confirm the current information in your medical records. Is it OK if I record that on the tablet?

Mrs Richards: No, that's fine, I knew that you would be asking some questions, but didn't you ask me those last week?

HcP Meg: Yes, I just need to clarify a few things. What's your current address?

Mrs Richards: Oh, I moved. So I am actually now living at Dingo Street, Downtown, number 24.

HcP Meg: Um. Oh yeah, that's different from what it was before.

Mrs Richards: Oh, yeah. There's like 32 stairs that you've got to walk up to get in the house and to get out of the house. So we've moved down to the lower ground level, which is heaps better.

HcP Meg: OK, that's understandable! Glad it's better for you. And is your phone number the same?

Mrs Richards: Oh, my mobile number's the same, but my landline has changed.

HcP Meg: OK. Can you please confirm both your landline and your mobile numbers, please?

Mrs Richards: My mobile number is still the same. My landline number is 795 3629.

HcP Meg: OK, thank you. Can I ask about your blood pressure? Are you still taking the same medications each day?

Mrs Richards: Yeah I am, my blood pressure's going well, but my specialist mentioned that my macula was getting worse and he was wondering if it was the blood pressure medication that was causing it.

HcP Meg: Oh OK, um all right um, there's nothing about your macular degeneration here in the medical records, um, which eye was it?

Mrs Richards: It's my right eye.

HcP Meg: OK. There's nothing about that here in your medical records, I'll just add that in there. And how long have you had that?

Mrs Richards: Ah, for about a year – I see the specialist monthly to get treatment for that.

HcP Meg: Has anything changed since we met last week?

Mrs Richards: Um, I'm actually able to move a bit more. So that's been really good. I can put my arm behind my back now and I can also lift my arm up, but not all the way up.

HcP Meg: Excellent. Um. OK. And how painful is your arm at the moment on a scale from 1 to 10? You said 9 last time I asked this question.

Mrs Richards: It's about a 7 now.

HcP Meg: Oh, that is an improvement.

Mrs Richards: Yeah.

HcP Meg: That's exciting. Can I just confirm which is your dominant arm, I don't feel like I …

Mrs Richards: It's my right arm. Unfortunately. It's the one that's got the injury.

HcP Meg: Mm, um, right, and is there anything you have been able to do this week, that you weren't able to do last week?

Mrs Richards: I can actually turn the kettle on. And I've got a Home Care nurse that comes and helps me shower and dress.

HcP Meg: OK. Fabulous! Would you like to set yourself some goals for next time we meet?

Mrs Richards: Ah I'm not really keen on goals. I just, if I don't achieve them then I get really, you know, disappointed with myself, so …

HcP Meg: Yeah, understand that – it can be difficult when things don't happen as planned. However, you, I think you'd feel a real sense of achievement when you achieve the goals that we set, even if it takes longer than expected.

Mrs Richards: Mm, I'll think about it if that's OK.

HcP Meg: Fabulous, we can come back to that next week when we meet.

Mrs Richards: Mm. Oh, I nearly forgot, I actually can't come next week, because I'm going away with my husband.

HcP Meg: Oh, lovely.

Mrs Richards: Yeah.

HcP Meg: And are you driving somewhere?

Mrs Richards: Um no, my husband will drive, but I was just wondering when am I going to be able to drive? Will it be very long?

HcP Meg: You can drive when you can reach your arm to the level of the steering wheel. That will depend on your level of improvement. Have you been doing your exercises four times a day?

Mrs Richards: Um, I do them in the morning, and sometimes in the afternoon, but I'm just so tired at the end of the day, I just can't.

HcP Meg: OK, cos you need to be doing them in the afternoon and the evening as well. Have you tried having a nap in the afternoon to help you do them in the evening?

Mrs Richards: No. I can't have naps, I've got kids and grandkids coming all the time and I'm too busy.

HcP Meg: OK, well, it's really important for your progress that you do do the exercises.

Mrs Richards: I'll try, yeah. Like I said I'm really busy, but I will try.

HcP Meg: I understand that you're busy and that it's tiring recovering, but it's really important that you do your exercises. Without doing your exercises we are not going to see the progress that we need for you to continue to improve.

Mrs Richards: I'll try and find a way that I can do the exercises more.

HcP Meg: Fabulous. Well, time's passing, let's begin your treatment for today.

Mrs Richards: OK, thank you.

CHAPTER 3

Mrs Richards' story

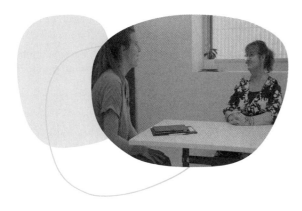

Healthcare Professional (HcP) Meg: Well, Mrs Richards, we appear to have five minutes left today and you seem to be doing well.

Mrs Richards: You think so?

HcP Meg: Yeah, you're certainly doing more with that injured arm this week than you were last week and you seem more engaged and happier, which is great.

Mrs Richards: Thank you.

HcP Meg: You are achieving those goals we established when I first saw you to help you feel less depressed and under-motivated. Think about what you have done today – that you could not do last week and tell me what you have done.

Mrs Richards: Well, I can lift a cup of tea and drink from it, which is nice and oh, I opened the door for the first time today, with my injured hand, so that's the first time I've been able to do that.

HcP Meg: Exactly, and you're also able to unbutton your jacket and put it over the chair using both hands. I don't remember seeing you do that either before. What about work. Um, what have you done in the last week that you've had difficulties doing before?

Mrs Richards: I can pretty much do most everything that I've done before, I'm just a lot slower than what I was. Um, I'm not getting as emotional as what I was either, so if there's something that someone asks me to do that I can't do, I just let them know that, you know, I can't do it or I get someone to help me. So that's been nice not being so emotional. I don't like the fact that I still can't drive to work though, but my husband likes that he can take me to work without the kids, so we get to talk. So that's nice.

HcP Meg: It's great that you're able to basically do everything required at work. Yes, driving will still happen – sooner than you think, I suspect – and you may miss the time spent with your husband! You've certainly been achieving all the goals we've established for the first week we've seen each other. You must be practising those movements and exercises the physio gave you, at home. And I suspect you're also trying to use your arm. Well done!

Mrs Richards: Thank you.

HcP Meg: You also seem to be less depressed and unmotivated than you were previously. This is great because we only have two more sessions scheduled.

Mrs Richards: Two more weeks, wow. I don't know what – what am I going to do, if I lose control of my emotions again?

HcP Meg: You're doing really well – and we can check in with the physiotherapist next session if you'd like, to reassure you about your improvement.

Mrs Richards: Well, I haven't been getting so overwhelmed and emotional as what I was before and if I see something that I can't do, I just keep telling myself, 'Do those exercises, do those exercises and you'll be able to eventually do it'. That helps me get further and further. So that's been good.

HcP Meg: Well done, that's quite an improvement. Mrs Richards, you're doing so well. And when we check in with the physiotherapist, they'll be able to reassure you of how much you've improved.

Mrs Richards: Cool. That's great.

HcP Meg: And now tell me, have you been sleeping?

Mrs Richards: When I get to sleep, I sleep really well – but getting to sleep, it takes like over an hour some days, so I wake up really frustrated.

HcP Meg: Oh, OK, that does sound frustrating. That is something we can work on in the next two sessions if you like. We had planned for 10 weeks depending on your improvement and you certainly are improving to the expected level of control of your emotions and also your overall mood – not to mention the use of your hand.

Mrs Richards: I've really enjoyed our sessions. So what will I do if I start losing control of my emotions again or I can't do things? What do I do then?

HcP Meg: Well, let's think about the next two sessions. So we'll have the hand therapist come and assess your ability and they'll take up 30 minutes of our session next week. So, what would you like to do in the remaining time in the last session?

Mrs Richards: Maybe something to help me sleep better?

HcP Meg: We can certainly work on that.

Mrs Richards: That'd be great.

HcP Meg: We'll see you next week for those sessions.

Mrs Richards: That would be great. Thank you.

CHAPTER 4

Exploring Reflection PowerPoint slides

Slide 2

Exploring reflection is really important in achieving effective communication in healthcare. Very important. The thing about reflection is that it is a conscious exploration, and it explores and clarifies the reasons for or possible causes of both satisfactory and unsatisfactory interactions. It can occur during an interaction or after. And what it does is it identifies why or why not an interaction was satisfactory or unsatisfactory. I think understanding is really important. It facilitates understanding both for the healthcare professional and those around them of the possible causes, sometimes immediate causes within an interaction and sometimes causes that occurred before the interaction and sometimes much earlier in a Person's life.

This enablement can bring about changes and achieve effective communication. And that not only provides effective communication, it ensures positive outcomes and meaningful interventions in the future. Very important in healthcare.

Slide 3

Yeah, we all need to learn and grow, don't we? It's something that's really important. So learning about ourselves, by exploring and clarifying the reasons for particular responses – for your own responses and sometimes for other responses – that can enable consistently for you to learn – and to achieve positive interactions. It can actually help you understand the reasons for your colleagues' reactions, and there might be various causes, sometimes related to the work environment and others for personal reasons. I think there's something about reflection that's really important, is that it helps us to learn about the Person that we're assisting or enabling. And they always experience negative emotions of some kind, often of the sense of vulnerability, disappointment, frustration and various other negative emotions. And it's really beneficial as a healthcare professional to be able to understand these emotions and to facilitate demonstration of empathy because of this understanding. The other thing that's really important in healthcare is service policies or guidelines. And one of the things about – they can really affect our responses in particular situations, but they develop for specific reasons, often from specific causes. So, it's really beneficial for healthcare professionals to be aware of these reasons and causes to ensure consistent conformity to the policies and the guidelines. Very important aspect of effective healthcare, but also of being appropriate within a health service.

Slide 4

Okay. Reflection is an interesting thing because some personality types are natural reflectors. Typically, they reflect about reasons why this happened, why it didn't happen within their daily events and within their life. However, there are other personality types that are totally unaware of reflection and they rarely do it naturally or automatically. The thing about reflection is that it may require commitment. Now being committed to reflection can be useful for those people who are not natural reflectors. This will require committing dedicated time to reflection. It can be very useful for those people who are not natural reflectors. Now one of the things that can help you develop your skills in reflection is using a model. Now there are various models, and I will discuss some models now. But you will need to find a model that suits you, that is suitable to your personality and the way you think.

Slide 5

So the first model is the Kolb learning cycle. Now this is a learning cycle, and people often say, 'Oh, it's a learning cycle; it's not a reflective –' Yes, it's true. It is a learning cycle, but it does encourage the development of skills in reflection. And each step leads to the following step, which creates a circle or a cycle. And it may suit your personality in a way that the others may not. So, step one in the Kolb learning cycle is to act or to behave, to do. And so, you do something and then you reflect about it. You think about what, why, how, where. And that's step two. And then step three, you consider the process and the principles that guided what happened or that might need to be applied in future interactions to guide future interactions to achieve really positive outcomes. And that leads to step four, which is you then plan and you return to step one and you act and behave. You do again. Okay. So, another model of reflection is the Boud, Walker and – Keogh and Walker. Now this is a different, quite a different model. It consists of three separate circles, and the circles are connected with arrows. So they're next to each other and there's arrows that point towards, backwards and forwards to each circle. Circle one considers personal experience, the behaviour, the feelings, the ideas. Circle two, you return to any event, you use positive emotions, and you remove controlling or negative emotions while evaluating and examining the intent – what was happening – and the knowledge that you can – you have or other Person might have about the interaction. And circle three develops – and that's the outcomes, the first two developing a new perspective. So, the first two then helps you with circle three develop a new perspective and that allows you to change behaviours to apply and to provide a commitment to future interactions that will become positive. So, the first one is your experiences, the second one is the actual reflective process, and the third circle is the outcomes. So, they're all very important parts of reflection. The Gibbs – well, why did we get two then? Sorry. The Gibbs 1988 cycle is – it's a reflective cycle and it has six steps. You describe the interaction in step one. Step two, you consider the feelings and the thoughts of the interaction. Step three, you evaluate the feelings and thoughts and you think about why, what, how. And so step four is analysing. Consider their sources, their why, what, how, their causes, their reasons. And step five is to make a conclusion about the interaction. And then step six is to develop an action plan to ensure positive outcomes in the future. Now the Fish, Twinn and Purr. Now if you look at the dates when these were all developed, they developed around a similar time, some were in different parts of the world, but they certainly – it was a time when people were understanding the need for reflection and, therefore, they also understood how difficult it could be for people who are not natural reflectors so they developed particular models. And the Fish, Twinn and Purr model has four strands, and they are combined to provide a framework of reflection. So, this first strand is the factual strand, and then you've got the retrospective strand which makes you think about what happened, the substratum strand and the connective strand. This is actually – the strands are complementary, they operate together, and they operate together in order to produce the best possible outcomes, and the most appropriate changes in thoughts, feelings and actions, so you have positive outcomes. The first two are the easiest ones to do, so that's the facts of what happens and retrospective why they might have happened and, you know, the results of those interactions. And they actually produce possibilities of, 'Oh, what can I do differently next time?' The last two produce much deeper reflection, and they sometimes are forgotten because they're a little bit harder to do, but this model has not got questions to answer. It's got a variety of things that – I don't know why that keeps coming and going.

Okay. The Johns structured reflection. Now, this is 2022. It's the 10th edition and it's simplified. This is a simplification of it. It's about reflection. And you begin with describing the experience, and then you consider the possible causes and any background information. What were the influencing factors, the aim of each action, and the possible reasons for the actions? Consider the consequences along with the resultant feelings that everyone might have experienced. And what could I have done to deal with it better? Why other actions were not chosen? Why didn't I do something different? Why didn't they do something different? What were the possible consequences of these other actions? And then you consider the resultant learning for future events. So, this is actually something that's quite important. Again, it's a model that well may suit your – your particular personality. Johns initially developed this in 2000, so it's been around for a long time and it's been used by many people, as have they all. Okay. Now the last model here is the O'Toole model, 2020. It's going – about to come out again in 2024, and we're going to look at it in a bit more detail in a moment. All these models of reflection will assist in developing the required skills to reflect, and that's something that's very important. Okay.

Slide 6

Now here it is, the healthcare-related model to guide reflective care. So, what you do is you choose to and you allocate time to reflect about your healthcare practice. And then you choose a challenging or interesting event. It may not be necessarily a challenging one, you may choose just something that was interesting that you really thought, 'Wow, that was interesting'. Then you describe and explore the chosen event. So, describe it, what happened. And there might be other things than just the people that are interacting, there might be other things in the environment that are happening. And then you think about all the reactions, both of yourself and of the Person. And sometimes there's more than one Person involved, so you need to think about that. You establish goals for similar future events or interactions that will ensure positive interactions. Develop strategies or action plans that will actually help you achieve those goals. And then you act in a way to fulfil the plans, reflecting upon and changing healthcare as necessary. And then, of course, you go back to allocating time to reflect again. And again, you move around, considering each of the events that you want to explore.

Slide 7

So, using reflection in practice can be very beneficial. It certainly will increase your awareness of yourself and awareness of the Person, which can be very important, not only, as I said earlier, in developing empathy and demonstrating empathy, but also in ensuring that you have most appropriate and effective outcomes. I think one of the things that's very good about reflection is it does help you become aware of your areas of strength. And that's something that's really important. A lot of people forget they have areas of strength. And sometimes the areas for improvement, there's a lot of talk about strength and weakness as well. I think I prefer to think about us having areas for improvement, and we all have them. And if you first identify your strengths, you can use your strengths to actually help you develop skills to improve in the areas that are not really appropriate. I think one of the things about reflection, too, is that it helps you to understand and to be honest with yourself, and to be honest with others as well, which can be very important, especially if you're referring to yourself. It can help you to be way more predictable, and that's something that is not going to be a waste of time because predictability for the Persons around us, whether they be the patients or the colleagues or the carers, it's really important that we are predictable for them all the time. It definitely increases your competence in communication and therefore in practice. And this is something that is essential if you want to be an effective communicator and an effective healthcare professional.

Slide 8

These references – refer to all of the things that were mentioned in the slide about the – in Slide 5 that talks about the different – that lists the different models. So, if you feel that in the description that any of these might suit you, then go and explore them more in this. So, thank you very much, and we'll finish the recording now.

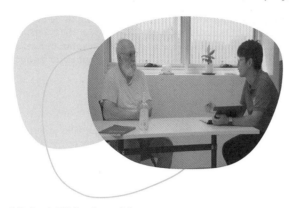

CHAPTER 5

Frank Bennet's story

Mr Bennet: Oh dear, I hope he's not my therapist, he doesn't look old enough to be out of school.

Michael: I'm looking for Mr Bennet.

Mr Bennet: (*Sarcastically*) Oh great – yeah, that's me.

Michael: Well, please follow me.

Mr Bennet: Oh, wonderful … Well, there are MANY other places I'd rather be than here, especially not sitting with somebody who should be still finishing school.

Michael: OK, Mr Bennet – I have worked here for five years and if you would prefer to see someone else, I think I can arrange that – but you need to wait at least one hour or more before you see them.

Mr Bennet: I can't wait for an hour and obviously you're older than you look so we should continue.

Michael: Well, Mr Bennet – tell me: why have you come here?

Mr Bennet: You've got the notes, so why don't you tell me?

Michael: The notes say you have injured your left arm. Is that correct?

Mr Bennet: Yes, I had a fall and I fell on my arm, and I hurt my wrist and it hasn't been getting any better. If I hold my wrist while I'm using it, it's a little bit difficult. Either I've got to use both hands at once or to use my left hand on its own.

Michael: Yeah, that would be difficult. But at least it wasn't your right arm you hurt.

Mr Bennet: Why do you say that?

There is a knock on the door.

Michael: Come in, the door is not locked.

Another HcP (HcP 2) enters the room.

HcP 2 Alex: Hello, good morning.

Michael: Oh, hi, Alex, I forgot you know Mr Bennet.

HcP 2 Alex: Nice to see you again.

Mr Bennet: Hi, Alex, it's good to see you.

HcP 2 Alex: How are you this morning?

Mr Bennet: Oh, I've been better.

HcP 2 Alex: Yeah, you were telling me that you had an injury with your dominant hand. Mustn't have been nice hurting your hand like that and not getting it looked at.

Mr Bennet: No, it hasn't got any better.

HcP 2 Alex: Well I'm very glad you took the initiative to get an assessment today.

Mr Bennet: Oh, Alex, I didn't take the initiative, my family made the appointment for me – yeah.

HcP 2 Alex: Ah, well, I am very glad your family made the appointment today, because you actually have the best therapist I know looking after you.

Mr Bennet: Oh, really?

HcP 2 Alex: I've also noticed that your clothes are still a bit worn and I remember you telling me your washing machine was giving you some trouble.

Mr Bennet: Yeah, well, that was the reason I was sort of running late this morning, and between not being able to dress myself so I'm wearing clothes like this, and I don't usually look like this, and I can't keep them clean cos the washing machine's broken. Yeah, it finally got fixed this morning, so it's been a bit bad.

HcP 2 Alex: Yeah, I know, I understand, I understand. Well, I better leave you to it. I'll hope to see you, Michael.

Mr Bennet: It's good to see you again.

HcP 2 Alex: And I hope to see you out and about, and not in here.

Mr Bennet: That would be good. That would be good.

Michael: Oh, so your left hand's your dominant hand and you hurt that. I'm so sorry I made a wrong assumption there!

Mr Bennet: It's OK.

Michael: And that explains why you were so uptight when I came into the waiting room – totally understandable. I'm sure it's a relief to have the washing machine working again.

Mr Bennet: Yeah, yeah, like I said to Alex, I don't really enjoy looking like this but there hasn't been much option. But now the machine's fixed I can get my clothes cleaned and if we can fix my wrist, I might be able to wear different clothes.

Michael: Yeah, OK. Let's start again. Nice to meet you, Mr Bennet. I'm Michael.

Mr Bennet: It's nice to meet you too, Michael. Please call me Frank.

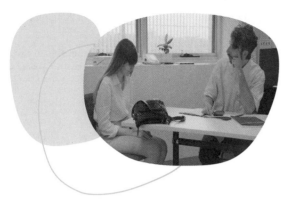

CHAPTER 6

Toni's story

Healthcare Professional (HcP) Glen: (*Looking at phone*) Good morning, Toni, how are we doing today?

Toni: I'm OK.

HcP Glen: (*Still looking at his phone*) Oh, that's good. Now, I just wanted to discuss some of the things that we were talking about last ... week. (*Looking up at Toni*) Um, Toni you don't appear to be OK, Toni. Is there anything happening? (*Looks back at phone*) OK, ah Toni, do you want to tell me what's going wrong?

Toni: (*Begins to cry*) Well, remember the last time I told you about my bird dying – the one that talked to me many times a day. Well, yesterday I took my dog, who is now my only company, to the vet. The vet does not think the dog will survive. It's too old. The vet will do their best to make him better, but the vet says that we will not be able to go out on our daily walk together any more. We both enjoy these daily hour-long walks together along the seashore.

HcP Glen: (*Looks up from phone*) OK, Toni, that is terrible, and yeah, of course you're very upset. Actually, did you want to tell me about what you were choosing to do with the bird cage and the toys you had for the bird? I think you said you were going to give them to your cousins (*Looking at his phone*) or ... might be looking forward to taking them?

Toni: (*Sobbing, shakes head*)

HcP Glen: No, OK. Look, Toni, I'm sorry, I'm just a little bit preoccupied today. Would you mind if I put my arm around you to give you a side hug?

Toni: (*In between sobs*) Yes, that would be good, thank you.

HcP Glen: OK. (*Sits next to Toni, puts his arm around Toni's shoulder, while looking at his phone*) Yeah, how you feeling now, Toni?

Toni: Thank you.

HcP Glen: That's good. That's very good to hear. (*Moves back to original seat and nods head flicking between Toni and phone*) Now, I know this would be very difficult for you to lose another one, or potentially lose another one so close, it's very troubling for you.

Toni: It has been a very distressing few weeks.

HcP Glen: (*Looks at Toni but then back at phone*) Yeah, look, now I realise that those things would have been very difficult, Toni, but your health and your ability to look after yourself is of course very important. OK, so have you been able to do anything we talked about last time you were here?

Toni: No, not really, it's been very difficult to do anything.

HcP Glen: (*Firmly*) No? OK, well I realise that those things have been very difficult, Toni – but it is very important that you look after yourself. You need to be doing these things every day, OK? Do you understand that?

Toni: (*Begins to cry again and nods*)

HcP Glen: Have you ... can you remember anything that we talked about?

Toni: (*Still crying, shakes head*)

HcP Glen: All right, well I'm going to get you a printout copy of what it is that we need you to do. Are you right if you just wait here for a few minutes while I go and get that?

Toni: (*Still with the occasional sob*) I'll be OK while you're gone. (*Toni continues to cry with her head in her hands*)

Seven minutes pass, with Toni sitting alone crying and waiting. Toni then stands up and moves towards the door.

HcP Glen: (*Returning*) Sorry, where do you think you're going? I told you that I was going to get the printout. I wasn't that long. Sorry that we had to find an electronic one and print that out. We didn't have any more paper copies left. So why don't we sit down, and we can talk about what it is that we are going to be going over the next few days, OK?

Toni: (*Unhappy but firm*) Actually, you were gone for more than five minutes, and I need to go the toilet.

HcP Glen: I'm sorry. I didn't realise I was gone that long. Do you know where the toilet is?

Toni: Yes, I do know where the toilet is, and I'll try not to be too long.

HcP Glen: OK. Do you need any help?

Toni: No, thank you.

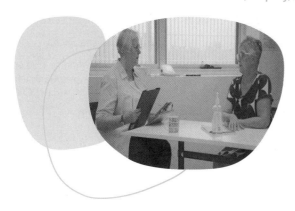

Chapter 7

Mrs Stein's story

Healthcare Professional (HcP) Pat Bates: Good morning, Mrs Stein. Oh, sorry I'm a bit late. I've been pretty busy.

Mrs Stein: Oh, I'm glad you're finally here; I was starting to think I had the wrong time or even the wrong date …

HcP Pat: No, no, no, no, not at all. OK, today I want to confirm my understanding of what we talked about last week.

Mrs Stein: Oh, OK, well we were discussing–

HcP Pat: (*Interrupting*) How've you been this week?

Mrs Stein: Well, I've been experiencing more–

HcP Pat: (*Interrupting*) Oh, before I forget, what was the number of that organisation that helps you with your homecare?

Mrs Stein: (*Sighing*) Oh, Homecare – oh, I know you want the number, I brought the card. (*Finds the card*) Um, and the number is 0427

HcP Pat: (*Writing*) 0427

Mrs Stein: 321 456.

Pat's phone makes a noise.

HcP Pat: Oh, sorry, I have to respond to this now, cos it's about what I am doing tonight.

Mrs Stein: (*Quietly*) Oh, why am I even here – this healthcare professional is just not interested in me.

Pat responds to the message and then puts the phone back on the table.

HcP Pat: Yeah, OK now.

Mrs Stein: Well, we were discussing ways of–

HcP Pat: (*Interrupting*) Ways to reduce your stress, I remember now. No, ways of doing your groceries, that's right. And I suggested a variety of things, you remember?

Mrs Stein: No, actually we were discussing how to reduce my–

HcP Pat: (*Interrupting*) No I remember, ways to reduce the number of times you have to come for treatment. That's right.

Mrs Stein: (*Impatient*) No, ways of reducing … my *pain*.

HcP Pat: Oh, your pain, oh, I remember now. That's right, I suggested a few different things though, didn't I? Things like doing those exercises to strengthen your muscles; using hot packs and positioning yourself very carefully when you're sitting, and when you're lying, that's really important. So how's your pain been this week?

Mrs Stein: Well, I tried to tell you that at the beginning of the session, it's much w–

HcP Pat: Better?! Oh, that is so good. (*Picks up phone and looks at it through interaction*) What do you think has made the difference?

Mrs Stein: Well, absolutely nothing!

HcP Pat: Nothing?

Mrs Stein: I have experienced much more pain this last week.

HcP Pat: (*Still looking at phone*) Oh, great. Now, what were we going to do today, can you remember?

Mrs Stein: Well, I'm not really sure, you didn't tell me. But how about we discuss ways of reducing my pain?

HcP Pat: Well, you do need to really start doing less and resting your body more, you know that, don't you? And also have you thought of ordering your groceries online and having them delivered?

Mrs Stein: We have discussed this. Can't you remember why I am unable to do that?

HcP Pat: No, I don't remember. (*Picking up tablet and scrolling*) Let me check your notes, I am sure that I will have recorded that.

Mrs Stein: (*About to speak but interrupted by a knock on the door*)

Another staff member opens the door.

Other staff member: (*To Mrs Stein*) Sorry to interrupt. (*To Pat*) Just wondering if you've got the notes, the notes from the meeting we had, the boss is looking for them.

HcP Pat: Oh, … oh, the notes from the meeting. OK, let me just … I'll be back in a minute. (*To Mrs Stein*) Sorry.

She leaves the room.

Mrs Stein: (*Aloud to herself*) I was hoping that this week would be different, they just don't listen. And here they've got me sitting here waiting unnecessarily. They could have finished the session and then go and look for their notes! Oh, my goodness.

A few minutes pass.

HcP Pat: Sorry about that, I had saved them, but I was very busy that I didn't call the right file name, so they couldn't find them. Sorry about that.

Mrs Stein: Well, maybe you should practise *listening*!

HcP Pat: (*Surprised tone of voice*) Do you think so? I thought I was OK at listening. Oh … Oh. Anyway, what were we doing? (*Looks at her watch*) You know you need to find ways of reducing the strain so that that will decrease your pain. You know that?

Mrs Stein: (*Nodding in agreement*) Look, we've discussed it and you know it's impossible in my situation.

HcP Pat: Oh? Can you remind me of your situation? Sorry.

Mrs Stein: We've discussed this over and over again.

HcP Pat: (*Talking over top*) We've discussed it … oh yes, that's right, we have discussed this – you are right. You live with your disabled sister and just a few weeks ago, your husband had a fall, didn't he? And he's not doing very well.

Mrs Stein: Yes, you finally remember something relevant about me!

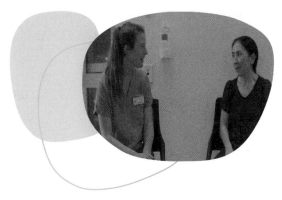

Chapter 8

Kim and Charlie's story

Charlie rushes into the waiting area and runs to the health-care professional (HcP) Pat (hugging her legs).

Healthcare Professional (HcP) Pat: Hello, hello. (*Returns the hug*)

Kim (parent): (*Anxiously*) Hi, I assume you're Pat?

Pat (HcP): Yes

Kim (parent): Sorry, sorry we are late. Our car is in a two-day service and we didn't expect to come here, so …

Pat (HcP): (*Shaking hands*) Nice to meet you.

Kim (parent): Nice to meet you too.

Pat (HcP): It's fine, don't worry – these things happen in life, don't they?! You're looking pretty tired and upset. Would you like to sit for a moment? (*Pointing to a chair*) But before you do, I just want you to meet – (*Turning to the HcP behind her*) This is Meg, who you'll be seeing today. OK? Before I go with Charlie, we'll go off and have some fun, we've got some fun things to do, haven't we? (*Charlie jumps up and down showing excitement*). Yeah, OK, so we'll see you later, OK? (*Pat and Charlie leave*)

Meg (HcP): Come and have a seat.

Meg and Kim sit together.

Kim (parent): Oh, thank you.

They sit for a moment.

Meg (HcP): What a morning.

Kim (parent): Ah, it's just so nice to sit down and relax a little bit, I just can't think clearly when I'm so stressed.

Meg (HcP): It's all right, take your time. (*Meg waits until Kim appears to be a little less stressed*) All right, are you ready to head over to the consultation room?

Kim (parent): Yeah. Thank you.

Meg (HcP): OK, let's go. It's just over here. Come in and take a seat.

Kim (parent): Thank you.

Meg (HcP): Is that chair comfortable for you?

Kim (parent): Yes, thank you. Is it me or is it quite hot in here?

Meg (HcP): Yes, it is a bit, would you like me to open a window?

Kim (parent): Yes, please. Thank you.

Meg (HcP): If that gets glary and we need to fix it, just let me know. All right, so Pat was wanting me to ask you about Charlie. Has there been any improvement with Charlie at preschool?

Kim (parent): Luckily, Sam and I have been talking about this regularly – so I can give you our combined thoughts. Certainly, some things have improved at home. Things at preschool seem to fluctuate. The 'culture' (I mean the habits and values) of the pre-school and their expectations are different to ours and Charlie has had a bit of difficulty adjusting to the differences. For example, we take our shoes off and put slippers on when we enter the house – the preschool only allows the children to take their shoes off when they're jumping on the trampoline. Of course, the trampoline is always supervised – and Charlie loves trampoline. We have one at home – which is used often by kids and sometimes adults! However, the keeping shoes on when entering the building is something Charlie is finding difficult.

Meg (HcP): (*Looking directly at Kim*) Different expectations in different environments can be difficult for children, especially when they're young. Is there anything else causing issues for Charlie when she's at preschool?

Kim (parent): (*Thinking and nodding to indicate 'yes'*) Again related to differences in habits or cultures. We always give thanks for food before we eat it – so Charlie will not begin eating until someone gives thanks for the food. This has caused frustration for the staff, but also for Charlie who has been kicking and hitting when the staff insist Charlie begins eating without saying thank you for the food.

Meg (HcP): Has this been explained to the staff at the preschool?

Kim (parent): (*Nodding yes*) Yes, we have talked to the staff, asking if they could allow Charlie to say thank you for the food, before beginning to eat. That has helped a little. If they have casual staff, however – they are often not told about it and thus there can be kicking and hitting!

Meg (HcP): Oh, that's very difficult to manage. Have you done anything to help the staff accommodate this need for Charlie?

Kim (parent): (*Nodding yes*) While Charlie has been more controlled at home because of the home program – so there is less kicking and hitting than previously – this has not happened consistently in the social setting of the preschool. We have tried to explain to the staff, and while some appear to understand, others just think Charlie should have more emotional control, regardless of the stimulus or the situation.

Meg (HcP): Mm, that is not unusual. Does Charlie have any friends at the preschool?

Kim (parent): (*Thinking*) Good question. I am not sure – we haven't received any birthday party invitations – although Charlie's birthday is soon, and we are sending invitations to all the children in Charlie's class at the preschool – so I hope we will know then by the children who come to the party and how they react to Charlie, if they like Charlie.

Meg (HcP): Well, I hope the party goes well and Charlie doesn't find any reason to hit or kick to express her frustration.

Kim (parent): (*Nodding in agreement*) Yeah, we'll see. We have discussed how to manage it if it does happen – and the discussions between Sam and Pat have certainly given us some ideas of how to manage any outbursts.

Meg (HcP): Pat tells me that your parents live with you. How do they go with managing Charlie's behaviour?

Kim (parent): They have particular expectations of children (seen but not heard!) so it can be challenging at times. Charlie loves having them at home with us, they often read to or play with Charlie when the other kids are doing their homework or playing games Charlie is too young to play. However, when they disapprove of any of Charlie's behaviour, Charlie becomes extremely distressed due to their disapproval.

Meg (HcP): It's good that they engage with Charlie, however difficult for both them and Charlie when they get negative responses.

Kim (parent): Yes indeed. You know it is really good to talk with someone other than Sam, about all this, thank you.

Meg (HcP): You're welcome.

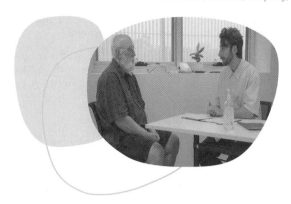

Chapter 9

Vic's story

Healthcare Professional (HcP) Glen: Hi, Vic, my name is Glen. I've heard you prefer to be called Vic, is that correct?

Vic: (*Wiping tears from eyes with a handkerchief*) Yes, yes, please call me Vic.

HcP Glen: OK great. Well, I'm seeing you today because my colleague who normally sees you is currently away, this week. But they will be back next week for you.

Vic: Are they OK?

HcP Glen: (*Looking directly at Vic and smiling*) Yes, they are doing OK, but thank you for asking.

Vic: (*Relaxing a little, but still wiping his eyes*) OK. So, what are we doing today?

HcP Glen: Well, I have been looking over your notes, and we will be doing what you normally do whenever it is that you come in. (*Looking directly at Vic*) Are you feeling OK today, Vic?

Vic: I'll be OK, in a minute. The last few weeks have been pretty difficult.

HcP Glen: That's all right, we all have very difficult times. It can take a long time to recover and it can [depend] very very much on the individual. What we've been noticing is that you've been coming in upset for quite a few weeks now.

Vic: Yeah, the records will show that I've been coming for treatment for quite a while.

HcP Glen: Is there anything in there that you would like to talk about?

Vic: (*Firmly*) Um, do you really want to know?

HcP Glen: (*Looking directly at Vic*) Yes, I would be interested in how you've been doing and what's been going on with your treatment. I'd also like to know what might have been causing some of this distress. Why you might have been feeling so upset for the last few weeks.

Vic: Well, I've been upset for a few weeks, sometimes more upset than other times. But the last few weeks have been very difficult. Most people, they understand and they let me cry, your colleague tells me that the treatment's really important and that um getting upset won't make the treatment go any easier. Your colleague tells me to stop crying and stop worrying about whatever's causing the tears, that I'll recover from whatever's happening, just forget about it and get over being upset and concentrate on the treatment.

HcP Glen: I'm very sorry that he's been saying those sorts of things to you. As I said very different events in your life can cause you to be upset and it can take considerable time to recover from for some individuals. And of course I'm sorry that you've been upset. Do you want to tell me what might have been causing your distress for the last few weeks?

Vic: (*Slightly relieved, wiping tears and controlling crying*) Oh, there was a car accident a couple of weeks ago and I lost my wife and my adult son, they were killed in the accident and I wasn't there, so I'm at home in an empty house.

HcP Glen: Well, that sounds very difficult for you, Vic. I'm very sorry and I am sorry that you haven't had the attention you needed for something like this.

Vic: (*Resignedly*) Well, at least it gets me out of the house. It's very hard being there, without them, um … at least, at least I know that I'll see them … I'll see them when I die. They're waiting for me. But it's very difficult.

HcP Glen: Yeah. Yeah, having that faith and allowing you to look forward to seeing them, it's very important. And I'm glad that it's comforting for you to know that you'll be seeing them um in the future.

Vic: This has been particularly helpful to talk to you now. Normally I'd talk to the minister at our church, normally I'd talk to him, but he's away.

HcP Glen: Well, we do have a chaplain here that you could spend time with if you would like. Um, that could be helpful to express some of your feelings and explore a bit more of your faith. Would you like to see them? I could set up a meeting.

Vic: Yeah, yeah, that might be helpful. That might be good.

HcP Glen: Good, I'll give them a ring now and see if we can set up some time for you.

Vic: Thank you, this has been much more helpful than I expected.

HcP Glen: Well, that's good.

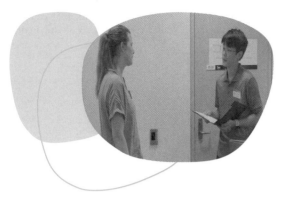

Chapter 10

Michael and Meg's story

Healthcare Professional (HcP) Michael: (*Leaving store-room*) Hi, Meg, I have just spent five minutes looking for a green and yellow snake in the storeroom. Any idea where it might be?

HcP Meg: Slow down. Tell me about that again.

HcP Michael: I really need a green and yellow snake to have an effective and successful session.

HcP Meg: There is a pink and purple snake, it's the same weight as the green and yellow snake, could you just use that?

HcP Michael: Yes, there is a pink and purple in the storeroom but, no, definitely no, because green and yellow snake is the favourite colour of the Person I'm seeing. It won't be helpful if I'm using the wrong colour.

HcP Meg: Oh, really, the green and yellow one isn't there? Wow, I'm sure that I returned it, although come to think of it, somebody did say that they were going to use it and take it off-site for a visit in the afternoon, and then bring it back in the morning as no one had it booked.

HcP Michael: I booked the green and yellow snake this morning! Which colour did you book?

HcP Meg: I booked a snake – but I didn't specify the colour! Weren't there two green and yellow ones?

HcP Michael: Yes, there are 2 green and yellow snakes, but one of them is being used by the team travelling outback in the remote area. Are you sure you heard that conversation about the green snake yesterday?

HcP Meg: Um … it could have been yesterday or it could have been the day before, I'll have to check my diary. I overheard something about the conversation of the snake in the storeroom, but I didn't really look at them because I was bent over looking for the weighted dog. And I only really saw the side of their face and I was trying to work out where Dotty was and they said that they'd left Dotty in Treatment Area 3 for me – I knew that I needed Dotty for the following session so I was going to move Dotty into the other treatment area room, I don't remember what it's called, it on the other side of the storeroom.

HcP Michael: Come on, Meg, the area you are talking about is Treatment Area 5.

HcP Meg: Come to think of it, Dotty might still be in Treatment Area 3.

HcP Michael: Meg, I know you are new here, but there are many things to learn, including the names of your colleagues along with where to return equipment to this storeroom, despite the labels! Can you remember who it was that said they had left Dotty in Treatment Area 3 and was going to take the green and yellow one?

HcP Meg: I'm not sure of their name and they weren't really looking at me – I only saw the side of their face! Doesn't someone keep track of who is off-site in the afternoons, can you not check the off-site register to find out …

HcP Michael: All right, that might help, I'll go and check the diary to see who had that late session. Mind you, I'm not sure that it will help me for this session now. I may need to try something else that has a similar weight. Who knows how accepting the little Person will be of a change – they typically do not manage well. Good luck with your session.

HcP Meg: Thank you.

HcP Michael: Will the pink and purple snake be OK for you and your little Person?

HcP Meg: Yes that will be OK, I can use that one. Yep. Although, I might still check Treatment Area 3. But I'll have to check that and let you know.

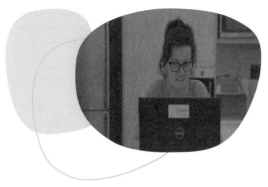

Chapter 11

Julien's story

HcP Meg: Good morning, Julien, sorry it took so long to connect today.

Julien: Gosh, that's OK. Thank you for ringing me to tell me though – I was beginning to wonder if perhaps I might have the wrong time, but then I remembered that you'd sent the invitation for this time, so I didn't have the time wrong.

HcP Meg: Yes, yes, well, I realised when we had trouble connecting and the technical officer who usually assists was with someone else, that I would be late! So that's why I needed to ring you.

Julien: Were you able to work out what the problem was with the connection?

HcP Meg: It seems that we have a new internet supplier and there were some unexpected issues they needed to solve. I don't think they expected as many of us to be on the internet every day.

Julien: Yeah, we sometimes have difficulties connecting if it gets windy, and they can't seem to explain why. But anyway we're connected – that's the main thing.

HcP Meg: Yes, that's exactly right. So let's begin. Is it OK if I record the session?

Julien: Yes, yes, please go ahead.

HcP Meg: OK, so how have you been this week? Have you been able to do the exercises the physio suggested and those necessary activities now that you have the pieces of equipment provided by the occupational therapist?

Julien: Yes, I'm very pleased to say that the answer to both of those questions is yes! Um and I still have a little bit of pain – but I'm able to do the exercises three times a day – but I do have to take a break, so usually about a 5 or 10 minute break, um and then I can begin again.

HcP Meg: Fabulous! Can you show me how much movement you have in your arm now?

Julien: Yeah, I'd love to. Can you see me OK? (*She raises her arm above her head*) So, yeah.

HcP Meg: Yeah, just like that. That's fabulous.

Julien: (*Moving her arm across her body and placing her hand on her other shoulder – with a slight grimace on her face*) And then I can …

HcP Meg: Oh, there you go.

Julien: Yeah. It's not too bad! Yeah. (*Smiling after stopping moving*)

HcP Meg: (*Smiling*) Yeah, that's much better.

Julien: Yeah yeah. Thank you.

Meg: Now, can you please turn to the side and show me your arm moving backwards and forwards?

Julien: Yeah.

HcP Meg: Yep, just like that.

Julien: You can see OK? (*Julien turns away from the camera with the affected arm closest to the camera and moves her arm backwards and forwards*) So d'you just want me to go – (*there's some restriction in the backward movement*).

HcP Meg: (*Smiling and looking carefully while Julien moves her arm*) Yep, just like that. OK, all right. Thank you. Now would you mind standing up so I can have a look at your knee?

Julien: Yeah. (*Standing up, and moving back a little to allow Meg to see the knee, with the affected knee closest to the camera*) It's this one here. Let me know if you can see it. (*Lifting her knee to make a right angle at her hip and her knee*)

HcP Meg: Yep. That's it, that's good. OK. (*Meg watches Julien move her knee*) OK. All right. Your movements are smoother than they were and now you can lift it and bend it at a right angle.

Julien: Yes.

HcP Meg: You couldn't do that a few weeks ago.

Julien: I know, I think the exercises are really helping. Absolutely.

HcP Meg: Have you been practising the sit-to-stand exercise?

Julien: Um, yes, I have. Um, I've got to be honest and say that I know it will help me, um, but I kind of feel a little bit hesitant. I'm not feeling confident about that movement. I'm just afraid that it's going to produce a little bit too much pain in my knee when I stand.

HcP Meg: Yep, yeah, that's understandable, however the sit-to-stand exercise will help you develop your ability and your confidence that you need to stand.

Julien: Yeah, that makes sense.

HcP Meg: How are you going getting dressed and going to the toilet?

Julien: Ah, yes, so the pieces of equipment that you've given me have been really, really helpful. I can dress myself now independently, I can even pull up my own undies and my long pants. Um, but I have to remember to dress … um I tend to dress the injured side first and that's helping my ability a lot to be dressing independently. I don't know, what do you think?

HcP Meg: Yeah, that sounds good. Um, what about going to the toilet?

Julien: Um, well, the raised toilet seat that you provided has made a huge difference. Absolutely life saver. As well as the shower chair that's hugely helpful as well. As you can imagine I wasn't very confident in the shower, so obviously that's a really difficult space, because it's slippery and wet and there's lots of things that could interfere with my stability, um I could fall and hurt myself on, um but it's working out really well. I am a bit slow – and that's been noted by the family. We do have two showers but it's just a matter of logistics, trying to make sure everyone can have their time, the time that they need in those areas. But I have been wondering, um when the tradie might come to install the rail, we talked about a rail.

HcP Meg: Actually, I'm not sure – but I can check for you. I'll email you through a possible date. The tradespeople we use are very good, but they're also very busy and so I'll have to let you know as soon as I know. Um, yeah, sorry about the delay.

Julien: That's fine. That would be great. Thank you so much, cos yeah, I worry about falling over in the shower – there is a little step, so again just to have that rail would help me feel a bit more confident.

HcP Meg: Yeah, that's so understandable – I'll give them a call and see if they can come to see you sooner if possible. The other thing that we need to check is how have you been sleeping? I saw in your notes that you have been having difficulty sleeping because of the pain. Has that improved now that the pain is less?

Julien: Yeah, well, thank you for asking – yes, as we talked about: sleep is so crucial to recovery and feeling strong enough to keep on with the exercises. But I must say I am finding it difficult to get a comfortable position when I'm sleeping, especially because I like to sleep, or I have in the past, I've slept on the side where the injuries are, so that's my natural go-to position. The pain has not been as bad, but what I have decided to do is, um just put some Panadeine and a glass of water beside the bed, so if I do wake up and I'm in pain, I can take the medication and that enables me to sleep through the rest of the night.

HcP Meg: That's good – it's good to hear that your sleep is improving. Sleep is so important for recovery.

Julien: Oh gosh, yes! Got to say, I also love the fact that the bed is higher. I can get in and out so easily and I feel so confident doing that, so that's really helpful. It's certainly made a huge difference. Makes it so much easier to get on and off the bed, which is logical, but yeah, a huge difference, so thank you for that one.

HcP Meg: That's also so good. It sounds like you're really improving. So you have another telehealth session with the physio in a few weeks and that means you must keep doing the exercises. Um, I'll write in your file indicating you've increased your range of movement in your shoulders and in your leg. But that your leg needs more ideas to increase the bend in it. You're making good progress and the physio will support you with that.

Julien: Yeah, OK, that's brilliant. Look, thank you so much. I really appreciate the call and being able to connect with you and just check in, that little reminder is encouraging particularly to focus on those exercises that I've sort of been ignoring a little bit. So thank you again. Thanks so much.

HcP Meg: You're welcome.

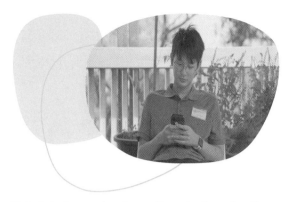

Chapter 12

Sadi's story

Please note this transcript has translated the 'text speak' that appears in the video and is not exactly as the text messages appear.

The following is a text conversation.

HcP Sadi: Just made it home. I'm sick of people telling me I am too young to be a qualified healthcare professional!

Friend 1 on Facebook Stephen: That's a compliment! Why be unhappy?

HcP Sadi: I've been working for 6 years. So what if I look young! Maybe I need to have my years working on my name tag!

Stephen: Relax, take it as a compliment!

HcP Sadi: Maybe you're right. But wait till I tell you what happened yesterday. I was talking to James Stevenson; you know, that news presenter. After he mentioned my age, I told him he was too old to be reporting the news! He laughed and said what a great reply!

Friend 2 on Facebook John: Wow, you have James Stevenson as one of your patients. Why? I thought I saw him last night reading the news.

HcP Sadi: Oh, you did, he has injured his knee so he can still present the news, provided he takes painkillers.

John: How did he hurt his knee?

HcP Sadi: Playing football. Tore his anterior cruciate ligament. He had surgery a few weeks ago. Now he's coming in for therapy until he recovers completely.

Friend 3 on Facebook Julia: Wow. Why hasn't that been reported in the news!?

HcP Sadi: When he came in yesterday he said he didn't want everyone to know, because he felt very stupid injuring himself.

Friend 4 on Facebook Tim: Hi, everyone, I just joined – are you talking about that cute guy who presents the news? I didn't know he played soccer!

HcP Sadi: Yep. He's a nice man – even though he thinks I'm too young to be a healthcare professional!

Tim: Yeh, I saw that – agree with Sado though – great compliment!

HcP Sadi: Maybe – but it happens so often, I'm over it!

Tim: Well, I don't agree with the comment about him being too old! I think he's young!

HcP Sadi: Yeah – just an angry me, third mention of my young appearance that day – he is nearly old – he's 34, turning 35 in a few weeks according to his DoB.

Stephen: What is DoB?

HcP Sadi: Date of Birth.

John: Wow! When's his birthday? We should send him Happy Birthday messages on the online chat connected to the news.

HcP Sadi: Great idea. DoB is 15/04/1997.